SAY NO TO
HEART
DISEASE

patrick
HOLFORD

SAY NO TO
HEART
DISEASE

piatkus

PIATKUS

First published in Great Britain in 1998 by Piatkus Books
Reprinted 9 times
This edition published 2010
Reprinted 2011

A CIP catalogue record for this book
is available from the British Library.

ISBN 978-0-7499-5348-5

Design by Paul Saunders
Illustrations by Jonathan Phillips

Typeset by Phoenix Photosetting, Chatham, Kent
Printed and bound in Great Britain by CPI Mackays, Chatham, ME5 8TD

Note from the author: In almost all cases heart disease is completely
preventable, and, provided you have not already had a heart attack or stroke
which has resulted in severe damage, completely reversible. This is what I
believe on the basis of the logic and evidence presented in this book.

Piatkus
An imprint of
Little, Brown Book Group
100 Victoria Embankment
London EC4Y 0DY

An Hachette UK Company
www.hachette.co.uk

www.piatkus.co.uk

Contents

ACKNOWLEDGEMENTS

This book would not have been possible without the support of Jan Shepheard, for taking care of things in my absence and putting up with the early mornings. On the research side, my thanks go to Anne McKeever, Information Officer at the Institute for Optimum Nutrition, my research assistant Pam Self, Antony Haynes for his help in researching insulin-resistance and permission to use the chart on page 48, and the many scientists who have helped me access the latest research. Finally, my thanks go to Natalie Savona for her editing and to Heather Rocklin and her team at Piatkus for their editorial advice, support, encouragement and assistance.

Guide to Abbreviations and Measures

1 gram (g) = 1000 milligrams (mg) = 1,000,000 micrograms (mcg or µg). Most vitamins are measured in milligrams or micrograms. Vitamins A, D and E are also measured in International Units (iu), a measurement designed to standardise the different forms of these vitamins which have different potencies.

1 mcg of retinol (mcg RE) = 3.3iu of vitamin A (RE = Retinol Equivalents)

1mcgRE of beta-carotene = 6mcg of beta-carotene

100iu of vitamin D = 2.5mcg

100iu of vitamin E = 67mg

1 pound (lb) = 16 ounces (oz)   2.2 lb = 1 kilogram (kg)

mg% = mmol × 38.7

In this book calories means kilocalories (kcal)

References and further sources of information

Hundreds of references from respected scientific literature have been used in writing this book. Details of specific studies referred to are listed on page 140. Other supporting research for statements made is available from the Lamberts Library at the Institute for Optimum Nutrition (ION) (see page 146). Members are free to visit and study there. ION also offers information services, including literature search and library search facilities, for those readers who want to access scientific literature on specific subjects.

HOW TO USE THIS BOOK

Heart disease is a complicated subject so I have structured this book to make it easy for you to understand what you need to do to keep your heart healthy. Part 1 explains the cardiovascular system, what cardiovascular disease is, and why you can expect almost complete protection by following the advice in this book. Part 2 describes the key new theories on major contributive factors to heart disease. Reading this section will help you to understand the basis for the practical recommendations later in the book. Part 3 tells you what the risk factors are, how to work out your own risk, and which areas of your diet and lifestyle to focus on in order to minimise your risk. Part 4 shows you the evidence for how nutrients and dietary changes can help you avoid heart disease, while Part 5 gives you clear, practical guidelines for staying free of it.

Medical advice

While, in truth, many of the strategies recommended here have proved more effective than conventional drug therapy, the recommendations in this book do not replace those of your doctor. If you wish to change your medication please consult your doctor.

PART 1

HEART DISEASE – THE MODERN EPIDEMIC

CHAPTER 1

FIRST THE BAD NEWS

One in two men *and* women die from heart disease.

Every year nearly 300,000 people in Britain die prematurely from a stroke or heart attack. One man in every four will have a heart attack before retirement age and a quarter of deaths occur in people under the age of 65. For women, heart disease and strokes are second only to cancer as the leading cause of death between the ages of 35 and 54. While heart disease usually strikes after 45, even by the age of ten fatty deposits (which herald the beginning of arterial disease) are already present in most people's arteries. So widespread is this modern epidemic of heart disease that we almost take it for granted. We fail to protect ourselves from a disease, the cause of which is largely known, and the cure for which is already proven. It is a more life-threatening disease than AIDS. According to the US Surgeon General, of the 2.2 million Americans who die each year, no less than 1.6 million die from diet-related diseases, predominantly of the heart and arteries.

There is nothing natural about dying from heart disease. Many cultures in the world do not experience a particularly high incidence of strokes or heart attacks. British people, for example, have four times as much heart disease by middle age as the Japanese. Autopsies performed on Egyptian mummies who died in 3000 BC show signs of deposits in the arteries but no actual blockages that would have resulted in a stroke or heart attack. Despite how obvious the signs of heart attacks are (severe chest pain, cold sweats, nausea, fall in blood pressure and weak pulse), in the 1930s they were so rare that it took a specialist to make the diagnosis. According to American health records, the incidence per 100,000 people of heart attack was zero in 1890. By 1970 it had risen to 340. Although deaths did occur from other forms of heart disease (including calcified valves, rheumatic heart and other congenital defects), the incidence of actual blockages in the arteries which cause strokes or heart attacks was minimal.

Even more worrying is the fact that heart disease is occurring in younger and younger people. Autopsies performed in Vietnam showed that one in two soldiers killed in action, whose average age was 22, already had atherosclerosis (deposits in the arteries). Nowadays most teenagers can be expected to show signs of atherosclerosis, which heralds the beginning of heart disease. Obviously, something about our lifestyle, diet or environment has changed radically in the last 60 years to bring on this modern epidemic.

TWENTY YEARS LESS HEALTHY LIVING

The cost of heart disease is, on average, 20 years less life. While the healthy human lifespan is at least 100 years, the vast majority of people die prematurely from heart disease or cancer. Even those who do reach their nineties are often not in good health, suffering from Alzheimer's or crippling arthritis. No wonder we sometimes ask, 'Who wants to live that long anyway?'

But you *can* be a healthy 100-year-old. Consider the cases of four pioneers of optimum nutrition. Dr Linus Pauling, twice Nobel prize-winner, discovered the value of vitamin C when he was 65 years old. He died at 93, having produced some of his most significant work after he turned 90. Dr

Roger Williams discovered vitamin B5 and folic acid and was actively teaching and writing until he was 95, dying at the age of 96.[1] Dr Carl Pfeiffer, who pioneered nutritional therapy for mental illness, had a massive heart attack at the age of 51. He was told that he would not survive without a pace-maker, and even then no more than 10 years. He changed his nutrition and lived to 80 years old, again active to the end. Dr Abram Hoffer, another optimum nutrition pioneer, discovered the value of vitamin B3 when he was 35 years old, and lived well into his nineties, writing, researching and seeing patients at the age of 80. All these people were middle-aged before they started to make real changes to their diet and lifestyle.

Yet one in five men and one in nine women now die of heart disease before they reach 75. If you can eliminate the risk of heart disease you can expect ten to 20 extra years of healthful living, assuming you don't die of cancer or spend your old age suffering from arthritis or Alzheimer's. However, the simple changes you can make to your diet and lifestyle to reduce the risk of heart disease, are also known to minimise your chances of suffering from these other debilitating diseases. Following the advice in this book will add years to your life, and life to your years.

CHAPTER 2

THE POWER OF PREVENTION

No disorder has been more thoroughly investigated than heart disease. Strangely, though, all the separate bits of information have yet to be compiled and presented as a clear preventive strategy. That is the purpose of this book – and you may be amazed to find that you can probably completely eliminate the risk of heart disease.

The chart below shows the major known risk factors (including medical statistics, all explained in later chapters) and the percentage decreased risk you can expect to gain by eliminating them. The good news is that you can get rid of all of them, except genetic predisposition, by making relatively simple, painless dietary and lifestyle changes.

What are the Risk Factors?

Eliminate these risk factors, through simple dietary and lifestyle changes, and you may reduce your risk by these percentages:

Medical Statistics	Per cent
High blood cholesterol (low HDL, high LDL)	60
High blood fats (triglycerides)	60
High blood pressure	30
High blood homocysteine	70

High lipoprotein (a)	50
Insulin-resistance	30
Diet	
Too much saturated fat	50
Too much meat	50
Too much salt (sodium)	25
Too much alcohol	50
Too little antioxidant vitamins C and E	50
Too little B vitamins	50
Too little potassium, magnesium and calcium	50
Too little essential fats (fish and seeds)	40
Too little fresh fruit and vegetables	30
Lifestyle	
Lack of aerobic exercise	50
Overweight	30
Smoking (20 cigarettes a day)	70
Too much stress	50
Genetic predisposition	5
Total risk reduction:	**100 per cent?**

These percentages are very approximate, based on current research. A good review of research and risk factors is 'Nutritional Aspects of Cardiovascular Disease', Department of Health, 1994.

Of course you can't really just add all the percentages together because many of these factors overlap, but the point is that if you were to do most of this you would achieve 100 per cent risk reduction. In other words, we already do know how to effectively eliminate the vast majority of risk factors for heart disease.

To illustrate this, let's say you are an average person with an average diet and lifestyle, and an average 50 per cent risk of dying from heart disease. Now you decide to eat more fruit and vegetables (rich in antioxidant vitamins, potassium, magnesium and calcium) and stop adding salt to your food. This will lower your blood pressure, reducing your risk by 30 per cent. Then you stop smoking 20 cigarettes a day, reducing your risk by another 70 per cent and decide to supplement your diet with vitamin C, E and B complex. The B complex will lower your homocysteine level (a toxin for the arteries), reducing your risk by 70 per cent. Vitamin C and E alone reduce risk by 50 per cent, and lower your cholesterol. Then you cut your alcohol consumption down to, on average, one drink a day, reducing your risk by 50 per cent, and start exercising three times a week, giving you another 50 per cent risk reduction. You also start eating more fish, such as salmon and tuna, and less meat. These fish provide essential Omega 3 fats and an associated 40 per cent reduction in risk. Just how far do you need to go before you have no risk at all?

In truth, we don't exactly know because studies haven't been done of the combined effects of all these proven preventive measures. The chances of virtually eliminating all risk are, however, very high indeed, even if you are genetically predisposed to heart disease.

CHAPTER 3

UNDERSTANDING BLOOD PRESSURE AND PULSE

Inside you is an amazing network of blood vessels which, if put end to end, would reach the moon! At their widest point these blood vessels are 2.5cm wide. At their narrowest point – the capillaries – they are only one-400,000th of a centimetre.

The cardiovascular system is made up of the heart and these blood vessels, which carry oxygen, fuel (glucose), building materials (amino acids), vitamins and minerals to every single cell in your body. Blood becomes oxygenated in the lungs where tiny blood vessels called capillaries absorb oxygen, and, in turn, discharge carbon dioxide, which we breathe out. The oxygenated blood is then fed into the heart which pumps it to all the cells. At the cells the blood vessels once more become a network of extremely thin capillaries through which oxygen and other nutrients pass. Oxygen and glucose are needed to make energy within every cell. The waste products are carbon dioxide and water, which pass from the cells into the capillaries.

The blood vessels that supply cells with nutrients and oxygen are called arteries, while those that carry away waste products and carbon dioxide are called veins. Arterial blood is redder because oxygen is carried by a substance called haemoglobin; this contains iron, giving it a red tinge. The pressure in the arteries is also greater than in the veins. As well as returning to the heart, all blood passes through the kidneys,

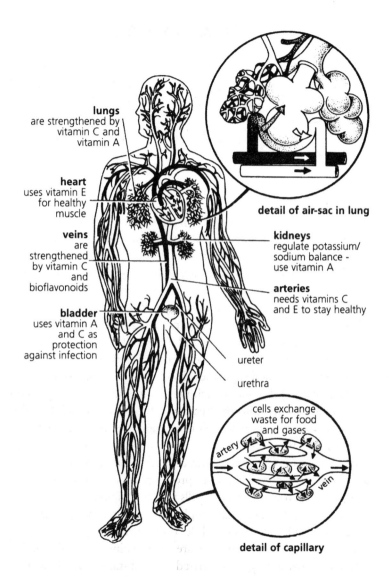

lungs
are strengthened by
vitamin C and
vitamin A

heart
uses vitamin E
for healthy
muscle

veins
are
strengthened
by vitamin C
and
bioflavonoids

bladder
uses vitamin A
and C as
protection
against infection

detail of air-sac in lung

kidneys
regulate potassium/
sodium balance -
use vitamin A

arteries
needs vitamins C
and E to stay healthy

ureter

urethra

cells exchange
waste for food
and gases

artery

vein

detail of capillary

Fig 1 – The Respiratory and Cardiovascular System

where waste products are removed and made into urine. This is stored in the bladder, ready for excretion.

WHAT CAUSES HIGH BLOOD PRESSURE?

One of the first signs of cardiovascular disease is increased blood pressure. Imagine a hosepipe attached to a tap that is turned on and off. The pressure is greatest when the tap is on, and lowest when the tap is off. That's what blood pressure is all about. A blood pressure reading of 120/80 means that the maximum pressure, just after a heartbeat, is 120 units; and the minimum pressure, when the heart is in a lull, is 80 units. Imagine if the hosepipe was metal rather than rubber. This would raise the pressure, wouldn't it? If the hosepipe was furred up, or if the fluid was thicker, these too would raise the pressure. So a raised blood pressure is a reliable indication that all is not right. Life insurance companies rely heavily on blood pressure to predict expected lifespan.

Approximately one in four people have high blood pressure, while only half the population have a blood pressure in the optimal range (below 120/80).

High blood pressure, also called hypertension, can be the result of any one of three main changes in the artery and is usually caused by a combination of these:

- **Increased constriction:** The blood vessels contain a layer of muscle. If this muscle contracts too much, the pressure increases. Smoking and stress can cause this kind of constriction, as can too much salt (sodium), or not enough magnesium, calcium or potassium, because these minerals control muscular contraction and relaxation.

- **Thicker blood:** If the blood is thicker or stickier this alone can cause small increases in blood pressure. The blood contains tiny plates, called platelets, which stick to each other. This ability to clot is what stops you bleeding to death if you cut yourself. If the blood clots too much, however, you run a greater risk of producing life-threatening blood clots, especially if the arteries are already narrow.

• **Atherosclerosis:** This means the narrowing of a blood vessel (due to damage and thickening of the blood vessel wall), often resulting in increased deposits of cholesterol and other substances. The blood vessel may also become less elastic, increasing the pressure.

IDEAL BLOOD PRESSURE AND PULSE RATES

A blood pressure of 120/80 or less is ideal. A top figure (systolic pressure) of more than 140, or a bottom figure (diastolic pressure) of more than 90, indicates a potential problem. A blood pressure of 150/100 indicates a serious risk of heart disease. For example, a 55-year-old man with a blood pressure of 120/80, will, on average, live to the age of 78. A 55-year-old man with a blood pressure of 150/100 is predicted to live to 72. High blood pressure, or hypertension, is a silent killer. Only one in ten people with raised blood pressure are aware of it. After the age of 25 most people's blood pressure increases quite rapidly. So a yearly blood pressure check is always recommended. If you're healthy there's no reason why your blood pressure should increase with age. Many primitive cultures show no such rise.

Low, Medium and High Risk Pulse and Blood Pressure Readings

	Low	Medium	High
Pulse	60–69	70–79	80+
Blood pressure	90/60 to 125/85	126/86 to 135/89	136/90 or higher

Your pulse rate (the number of times your heart beats per minute) is less a measure of the health of your blood vessels, and more an indication of the fitness of your heart. For example, a very fit cyclist may have a pulse rate of 40, while many people have a pulse rate of 80 beats per minute. So the cyclist's heart can get all the blood round with half the number of beats. His or her heart, which is essentially a muscle, is clearly stronger. The healthiest people have a pulse rate below 70 beats per minute. Interestingly, there is one lifespan statistic that is relatively consistent for all animals. We all have around three billion heartbeats in a lifetime. It follows that if your pulse rate were 80, you would have a lifespan of 71 years; if it were 60, 95 years. The better your diet and exercise regime, the lower your pulse rate will be.

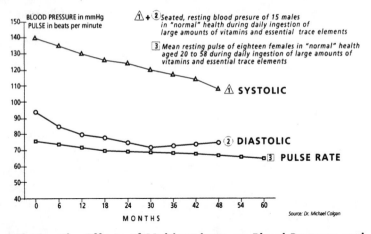

Fig 2 – The Effects of Multinutrients on Blood Pressure and Pulse

Both your pulse and blood pressure can be lowered with optimum nutrition. A three-month trial at the Institute for Optimum Nutrition in London, involving 34 people with high blood pressure, achieved an average eight-point drop in systolic and diastolic blood pressures, with the greatest decreases in those with the highest initial blood pressure.[2] In another study, Dr Michael Colgan found that people of all ages, when placed on comprehensive nutritional supplement programmes for five years, had gradual decreases in blood pressure, from an average of slightly above 140/90 to below 120/80.[3] Dr Colgan also found that their pulse rate dropped from an average of 76 to 65 over this time.

CHAPTER 4

UNDERSTANDING HEART DISEASE AND STROKES

Any disease of the blood vessels is called cardiovascular disease, popularly known as 'heart disease'. However, this is slightly misleading because cardiovascular disease can occur in the brain too, resulting in a blockage there which can cause a stroke. This is known as cerebrovascular disease (*cerebro* = brain). Blockages can also occur in the legs and other parts of the body, in which case they are known as thrombosis. But the most common site of blockage is in the coronary arteries which feed the heart itself with blood. This is called coronary artery disease. About half of all deaths from cardiovascular disease are from coronary heart disease and a quarter are from strokes.

The main life-threatening diseases are diseases of the arteries. Over a number of years changes can occur within the artery walls that lead to deposition of unwanted substances, including cholesterol, other fats and calcium. These deposits are called arterial plaque or atheroma, from the Greek word for porridge, because of their porridge-like consistency. The presence of arterial deposits and thickening is called atherosclerosis. Atherosclerosis occurs in very particular parts of the body, as shown in Figure 3.

Atherosclerosis, coupled with thicker than normal blood containing blood clots, can lead to a blockage in the artery, stopping blood flow. If this occurs in the arteries feeding any

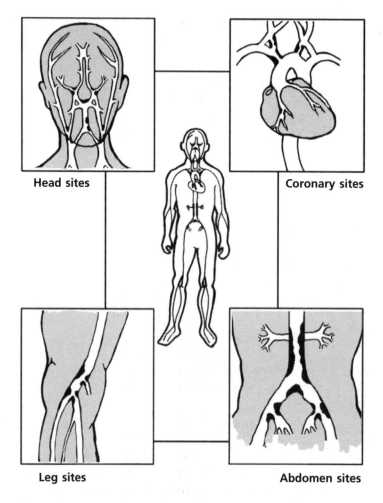

Head sites

Coronary sites

Leg sites

Abdomen sites

Fig 3 – Common Atherosclerotic Sites

part of the heart, that section of the heart dies from a lack of oxygen. This is called a myocardial infarction, or heart attack. Before this occurs, many people are diagnosed as having angina, a condition in which there is a limited supply of oxygen to the heart due to partial blockage of coronary arteries, characterised by chest pain, usually on exertion or when under stress.

If a blockage occurs in the brain, part of the brain dies, causing a stroke. The arteries in the brain are especially fragile and sometimes a stroke occurs not as a result of a blockage but because an artery ruptures. This is called a cerebral haemorrhage. If a blockage occurs in the legs this can result in leg pain, which is a form of thrombosis (a thrombus is a blood clot). When peripheral arteries become blocked this can result in poor circulation in the feet or hands and, eventually, pain and lameness. This is called claudication.

The popular misconception is that our arteries get blocked because we eat too much cholesterol. Although cholesterol does play a part in cardiovascular disease, it is now clear that there are a number of causes and several strategies for prevention. Part 2 explains the key factors that lead to cardiovascular disease and how to prevent them.

CONGENITAL DEFECTS

A small percentage of heart disease is caused by defects that are already there at birth. These are called congenital defects and may affect a valve in the heart or result in an artery that is too narrow. These defects cannot be corrected by changes in diet and lifestyle and may require surgical intervention.

PART 2

WHY HEART DISEASE? NEW BREAKTHROUGHS

CHAPTER 5

....

THE CHOLESTEROL MYTH

Back in 1913, a Russian scientist, Dr Anitschkov, thought he had found the answer to heart disease: he found that it was induced by feeding cholesterol to rabbits. What he failed to realise was that rabbits, being vegetarians, have no means of dealing with this animal fat.

Since the fatty deposits in the arteries of people with heart disease were also found to be high in cholesterol, it was thought that these deposits were the result of an excess of cholesterol in the blood, possibly caused by an excess of cholesterol in the diet.

Such a simple theory had its attractions and many doctors still advocate a low-cholesterol diet as the answer to heart disease – despite a consistent lack of positive research results. If the cholesterol theory were correct, we could expect that: people with high dietary cholesterol would have a high incidence of heart disease; raising dietary cholesterol would raise blood cholesterol; and blood cholesterol levels would be good predictors of heart disease.

PUTTING CHOLESTEROL TO THE TEST

Dr Alfin-Slater from the University of California decided to test the cholesterol theory:[4] 'We, like everyone else, had been convinced that when you eat cholesterol you get cholesterol. When we stopped to think, none of the studies in the past had tested what happens to cholesterol levels when eggs, high in cholesterol, were added to a normal diet.'

He selected 50 healthy people with normal blood cholesterol levels. Half of them were given two eggs per day (in addition to the other cholesterol-rich foods they were already eating as part of their normal diet) for eight weeks. The other half were given one extra egg per day for four weeks, then two extra eggs per day for the next four weeks. The results showed no change in blood cholesterol. Later Dr Alfin-Slater commented, 'Our findings surprised us as much as ever...'

Three other studies[5,6,7] also failed to find any increase in blood cholesterol levels when extra eggs were added to people's diets. In fact, as long ago as 1974, a British advisory panel set up by the government to look at 'medical aspects of food policy on diet related to cardiovascular disease' issued this statement: 'Most of the dietary cholesterol in Western communities is derived from eggs, but we have found no evidence which relates the number of eggs consumed to heart disease.'[8]

During the height of cholesterol phobia, Dr Jolliffe, renowned for his weight-reducing diets, started an 'anti-coronary club' and placed 814 men, aged 40 to 59, all free from heart disease, on a low-cholesterol, high-polyunsaturated-fat diet.[9] As a control group, he had 463 men of similar age and health status, who continued with a normal, and thus relatively high-cholesterol diet. Five years later, eight men on the low-cholesterol diet had died from heart attacks, compared to none in the control group! Ironically, Dr Jolliffe himself died from vascular complications of diabetes at the age of 59, so he never lived to see the results.

The Inuit people of North America were always an enigma with regard to the cholesterol theory. Their traditional diet, high in seal meat, has one of the highest cholesterol levels of any indigenous people's diet, yet their rate of cardiovascular disease is among the lowest. Other foods rich in cholesterol include shrimps. A more recent study from Rockefeller

University gave participants either three servings (300g) of shrimps or two large eggs a day, each providing 580mg of cholesterol. Researchers found that both groups had an increase in both the good HDL cholesterol *and* the less desirable LDL cholesterol (see next page), which they interpreted as meaning that neither diet significantly altered cardiovascular risk.[10]

It is now clear there is no strong relationship between intake of *dietary* cholesterol and incidence of cardiovascular disease. This said, however, a lot of high-cholesterol foods also happen to be high in saturated fat and may be fried. Such foods *are* associated with an increased risk of cardiovascular disease (a connection which is discussed more fully in the next chapter). It is therefore prudent not to go overboard on high-cholesterol foods, though, at the same time, there is no need for cholesterol phobia.

Switching from animal protein towards vegetable protein, especially soya, does significantly lower blood cholesterol and fat levels, thus reducing risk. These beneficial effects occur with as little as one serving of tofu or two cups of soy milk a day.[11] (For more on this, see page 109.)

GOOD AND BAD CHOLESTEROL

We have now learnt that cholesterol itself isn't the bad guy. After all, the body actually makes cholesterol itself and we all carry about 150g (one-third of a pound) of it in our bodies. Of this, 7g is carried in our blood. The body needs cholesterol to make sex hormones and vitamin D and to digest and transport fats (lipids). Nevertheless, having a high *blood* cholesterol level is associated with a doubled risk of cardiovascular disease. But it is the type of cholesterol in the body, and the way the body clears the excess from the arteries, that makes cholesterol relevant.

Cholesterol is made in the liver and should return there after it has been released (as a component of bile) into the digestive tract, where it helps digest fats before being reabsorbed into the bloodstream. Certain protein 'ships', known as low-density lipoproteins (LDLs), are responsible for carrying cholesterol *to* the artery wall; while others, high-density lipoproteins (HDLs), help to return cholesterol to the liver. So, if you have a low LDL cholesterol count and a high HDL cholesterol count, that

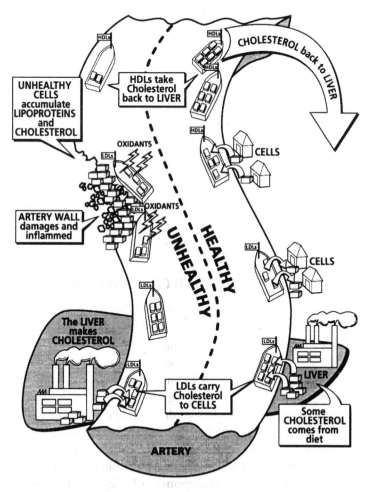

Fig 4 – How the Body Transports Cholesterol

is good news because it means that most of your cholesterol is on the HDL 'ship' which removes it from the arteries.

HDL cholesterol is sometimes thought of as 'good cholesterol' and LDL cholesterol as 'bad cholesterol'. Because of this, cholesterol tests now report not only your overall cholesterol level, but also how much of that cholesterol is on the 'good' HDL ship, and how much on the 'bad' LDL ship. If, for example, you have a high total cholesterol level and much of it is in the form of LDL, your risk is high. While, if you have a low total cholesterol level and much of it is on the HDL ship, your risk is low. This is usually reported as the ratio of total cholesterol to HDL cholesterol. If it's five parts cholesterol to one part HDL you have an average risk; if it's 8:1 you have a high risk; and if it's 3:1 you have a low risk.

IDEAL CHOLESTEROL LEVELS

Most laboratories report a 'normal' range for total blood cholesterol of between 120 and 330mg%. But, like blood sugar levels, so-called 'normal' cholesterol levels are based on people in average poor health. So what ranges exist in healthy people? This is the question Dr Emanuel Cheraskin and his colleagues set out to answer in a study on 1281 doctors, using an accepted health rating scale, called the Cornell Medical Index (CMI), in which the participants had to complete a questionnaire asking health-related questions. In the entire group, they found a range of cholesterol scores between 110 and 520mg%. The healthiest people (those with a score of 0 on the CMI) had cholesterol levels between 176 and 239mg%. In another study on dental students Cheraskin measured the effects of eliminating refined carbohydrates on the health of their gums. Those who achieved the best dental rating after the dietary changes had cholesterol scores in the narrow band of 190 to 210mg%. So this can be considered an ideal cholesterol range.

Low, Medium and High Risk Blood Cholesterol Levels

	Low		Medium		High	
	mmol/l (UK)	mg% (US)	mmol/l (UK)	mg% (US)	mmol/l (UK)	mg% (US)
Cholesterol	<5.18	<200	6.2	240	>6.7	>260
HDLs	>1.55	>60	1.16	45	<0.9	<35
Cholesterol/HDLs	3:1		5:1		8:1	

> = more than

< = less than

IMPROVING YOUR CHOLESTEROL LEVEL WITH NIACIN

One proven way to improve your cholesterol/HDL ratio (i.e. increase the amount of 'good' HDL and lower the LDL) is to take an inexpensive daily niacin (vitamin B3) supplement. This is a highly effective strategy (which also helps to lower another risk factor, lipoprotein (a), discussed fully in the next chapter). In one of the earlier studies on niacin, by Dr Grundy[12] patients given niacin had a 22 per cent drop in total cholesterol and a 50 per cent drop in blood fat level within a month! An appraisal of niacin in the *Journal of the American Medical Association* in 1986 concluded that it was 'the first drug to be used' when dietary intervention had failed to correct cholesterol statistics.[13]

Since the 1980s, two cholesterol-lowering drugs, gemfibrozil and lovastatin, have gained popularity among doctors due to their cholesterol-lowering effects. However, they are not nearly as effective as niacin in raising the beneficial HDL levels. In fact, niacin is, on average, five times more effective in raising HDLs, according to three recent US studies,[14,15,16] Another study, which combined niacin and gemfibrozil, found that, after four weeks, total cholesterol and LDL had decreased by 14 per cent, HDL had increased by 24 per cent, and the ratio of cholesterol to HDL had improved by 30 per cent.[17] That's enough to shift a person from the 'high risk' category to normal risk. What's more, triglycerides (blood fats) fell by 52 per cent. These results are consistent with those of other studies on niacin so it is likely that much of this improvement was due to the niacin rather than the drug.

There is one problem, however. At the level needed to produce these results (500 to 1500mg per day), niacin is a powerful vasodilator (i.e. it widens blood vessels), making you blush for about 30 minutes. This effect is not harmful. In fact it's beneficial but many people do not like it. By halving the dose, though, and taking it twice a day with food, the blushing usually lessens after a few days. An alternative is to take niacin inositolate, sometimes called 'no-flush niacin'. This is, however, not as effective in improving your cholesterol status and is best reserved for those who do not like the blushing effect of niacin.

Niacin has many positive effects on the cardiovascular system. Through its vasodilatory effect it improves circulation and may improve the elimination of excess cholesterol in this way. It also makes blood cells less sticky and therefore less likely to clump together, reducing the risk of a heart attack. It is certainly worth including in a prevention strategy for those with 'high risk' cholesterol figures.

THE DANGERS OF TOO LITTLE CHOLESTEROL

Since high blood cholesterol levels are associated with a high risk of coronary artery disease it is often assumed that having a low cholesterol level is good news. Not so, according to three independent research groups. One in Japan found that, while high levels are associated with cardiovascular disease (the incidence of which is low in Japan), low levels are associated with an increased incidence of strokes. As cholesterol levels dropped below 190mg% in a group of

6500 Japanese men, the number of strokes increased.[18]

Meanwhile, a Finnish researcher, Jykri Penttinen, has found a higher rate of depression, suicide and death from violent causes among those with very low cholesterol levels.[19] These findings were confirmed by David Freedman of the Centers for Disease Control in Atlanta who has found that people with anti-social personality disorders had lower cholesterol levels.[20] Freedman believes that people with very low cholesterol levels are more likely to be aggressive.

This suggests that cholesterol-lowering drugs should not be given to anyone unless their blood cholesterol level is high, even if they have cardiovascular disease.

HOW HEALTHY IS YOUR CHOLESTEROL?

Cholesterol is clearly an important substance in the body. There are dangers associated with having too much or too little of it, and whether it is in the form of HDL or LDL. And there is another factor: being a fat-like substance, cholesterol can be oxidised, or damaged, in the same way that oil paint is oxidised by air; when the lid is left off the can, the paint goes hard. Cholesterol can harden in a similar way. When this happens, it is more difficult for it to be transported around the body, and there is increasing evidence that this may be an important factor in cardiovascular disease.

The next question is: what damages cholesterol? The answer is oxidants, which result from smoking, fried food, pollution and normal body processes (including over-exercising and anaerobic exercise, such as sprinting during which the body goes into oxygen deficit because it's impossible to breathe in enough oxygen for the energy expended). On the other side are the body's protectors, the antioxidant vitamins A, C and E, plus minerals such as selenium and zinc. In truth there are hundreds of antioxidants in our food, especially in fresh fruit and vegetables. For example, in grapes you find proanthocyanadins, which is why a small amount of red wine may be mildly protective from heart disease, while too much alcohol is a well-known risk factor. Grape juice would be better. The antioxidant theory fits well with current research, which consistently shows a low risk of atherosclerosis among people with high intakes of anti-oxidant nutrients.

BEYOND HDL AND LDL CHOLESTEROL

The HDL and LDL 'ships' are special compounds made of fat and protein, called lipoproteins. Recently, scientists have started to investigate whether levels of these individual lipoproteins can help predict heart disease.[21] The lipoprotein that combines with cholesterol to produce the undesirable LDL cholesterol is called 'apoprotein B', or apo B for short. People with high levels of apo B also have high levels of LDL cholesterol and a higher risk of cardiovascular problems. The lipoprotein which combines with cholesterol to produce HDL cholesterol is called apoprotein A. (Actually there are two types: apo A1 and apo A2.) The higher your apoprotein A1 level, the lower your risk.

More recent findings, however, are also suggesting that the 'problem' fat may in fact be a much more specific and different kind of lipoprotein, not just LDL or indeed damaged cholesterol. Investigations into the fat deposits blocking vessels in people who had died from cardiovascular disease found a very high level of something called apoprotein (a) not to be confused with apoprotein A, which the body makes under certain circumstances. Apoprotein (a) has a natural tendency to attract lipids, binding with them to become lipoprotein (a), which readily sticks to artery walls. Levels of lipoprotein (a) are therefore highly predictive of cardiovascular disease. This is the basis of a remarkable new theory on a major underlying cause of cardiovascular disease and suggests an approach to its treatment which is further explained in Chapter 7.

....

CHAPTER 6

FAT FACTS AND FICTION

As scientists became disillusioned with low-cholesterol diets, they turned their attention to saturated fat, found predominantly in meat and dairy products. After all, eating too much fat leads to obesity and the incidence of heart disease in obese people is twice as high as in people of normal weight. Too much saturated fat raises levels of triglycerides (fats in the blood) and also blood cholesterol, both of which are good indicators of risk. The fatty streaks and deposits that occur in arteries are high in triglycerides, again pointing at fat as the culprit. In Western society, although not in some primitive societies, a high saturated fat intake is associated with increased risk of heart disease.

There is little doubt that eating too much saturated fat is a contributive factor in heart disease, but it is not the only one. After all, we know that the Inuit people of North America eat a high saturated fat and cholesterol diet based on seal meat and yet have one of the lowest incidences of heart disease, a mystery that will be explained later in this chapter.

FAT FACTS

Our bodies are composed of water (62 per cent), protein (22 per cent) and fat (14 per cent). We carry our water inside us, within cells that have a fatty 'skin'. Our nerves, which allow our 30,000,000,000 cells to communicate, are surrounded by a special fat to prevent them short-circuiting. Hormones and prostaglandins (chemical messengers in the blood) are made of fat. Half the brain is made up of fat. In fact, fat is essential for life – but not just any kind of fat.

Firstly, there are saturated and unsaturated fats. Saturated fats, like butter, lard, candle wax, coconut or animal fat, are hard at room temperature. The principal sources of saturated fat in our diets are meat, dairy produce and some kinds of eggs. While two-thirds of the calories in eggs come from fat, the kind of fat you find in an egg depends on what you feed the chicken. Battery chickens are often fed a high animal protein diet to promote growth, which also contains high levels of saturated fat. The fat in their eggs is therefore predominantly saturated. On the other hand, a free-range chicken is often fed grains, high in unsaturated fats, making their eggs high in these too.

Unsaturated fats, such as olive oil, sunflower oil and cod liver oil, are liquid at room temperature. The more unsaturated, the more liquid – and the more chemically active – they are. The trouble is that unsaturated fats go off easily, and turn rancid. You can taste this if you eat old nuts. This rancidity is caused by oxidation. It is the equivalent of a fat going rusty, just as metal does when exposed to oxides. High temperatures during cooking, especially frying, cause this to happen, as can keeping such fats for too long. Consequently, much modern processed food contains virtually no unprocessed, unsaturated fats because otherwise it would go off. This way, it lasts longer and is therefore a more profitable commodity. As a result, our diets are becoming poorer and poorer in these essential nutrients.

Incidentally, oxidised, damaged, or hydrogenated unsaturated fats (found in margarine and many processed foods) are as bad, if not worse, for you as saturated fats. Hydrogenating a polyunsaturated fat not only makes it saturated but also blocks the body's ability to use the good unhydrogenated polyunsaturated fats in nuts, seeds and fish. This means that fried food is bad news, especially if the food is high in fat, such as meat, eggs or cheese. On the other hand, a boiled free-range egg from a grain-fed chicken is a different story. Eggs also contain lecithin which helps the body to deal with cholesterol, though lecithin is again destroyed at the high temperature of frying.

THE FATS TO AVOID

Saturated fats primarily from land animals, such as pork, beef, lamb and dairy produce, are not a necessary component of a healthy diet and, in excess, increase your risk for cardiovascular disease. They make the blood stickier, and that, in turn, increases the likelihood of a blockage. You don't want too much fat in the blood either, because it encourages deposits and can become oxidised. Triglycerides (fats in the blood) are measured as an indicator of risk.

It is now generally thought that the level of triglycerides in the blood is not actually an underlying cause of cardiovascular disease, but rather a contributive factor that speeds up the process if arterial damage has already occurred. But there is an association between high triglyceride levels and high risk. Triglyceride levels can be high because we eat too much saturated fat, sugar and refined carbohydrate or drink too much alcohol.

Low Medium and High Risk Blood Triglyceride Levels

Low		Medium		High	
mmol/l (UK)	mg% (US)	mmol/l (UK)	mg% (US)	mmol/l (UK)	mg% (US)
<1	<89	1.5	133	>1.95	>173

> more than
< less than

THE FATS WE NEED

There are two 'families' of essential fatty acids. They must be included in our diet, as our bodies cannot make them. They are called 'Omega 3' and 'Omega 6' fatty acids. The 'grand-mother' of Omega 6 fats is linoleic acid. This can be converted into gamma-linolenic acid, or GLA, rich in evening primrose oil or borage oil.

The 'grandmother' of Omega 3 fats is linolenic acid. This can be converted into EPA (eicosapentaenoic acid) and DHA (docosahexaenoic acid) from which the very important and health-promoting 'prostaglandin series 3' fatty acids are made. These are strongly anti–inflammatory and protective for the heart and arteries.

We need both Omega 6 and Omega 3 fatty acids. Both are commonly deficient in the average diet, particularly Omega 3

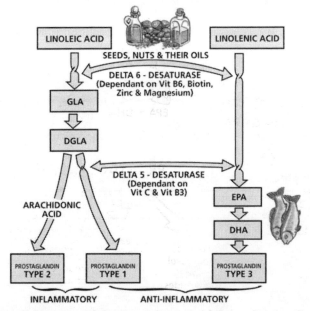

Fig 5 – Omega 6 and Omega 3 Fatty Acids

fatty acids. The best dietary source is seeds and nuts, together with vitamin E, the natural antioxidant protector. We need to eat these foods fresh to derive the benefit nature intended or, like the Inuit, we can learn the tricks of the food chain.

The Fat Food Chain

Fish get Omega 3 fatty acids by eating cold-water plankton. As these fish start to turn linolenic acid into EPA, they get eaten by carnivorous fish, like mackerel or herrings. These, in turn, concentrate more EPA, until they get eaten by a seal. Now we're talking concentrated EPA, which is what the Inuit get from their seal meat. Since seal meat isn't very appealing to most Western palates, the next best thing to have in our diet is carnivorous or oily fish, like salmon, herring, mackerel or sardines. The other alternative is to take a daily

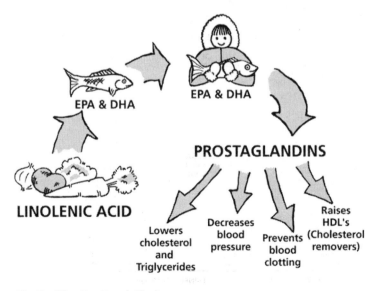

EPA & DHA

EPA & DHA

PROSTAGLANDINS

LINOLENIC ACID

Lowers cholesterol and Triglycerides

Decreases blood pressure

Prevents blood clotting

Raises HDL's (Cholesterol removers)

Fig 6 – The Fat Food Chain

supplement of concentrated EPA, which usually comes with some DHA and vitamin E, to prevent oxidation.

The Eskimo Enigma

This fat food chain also explains the enigma of the Inuit people. The traditional Inuit diet is among the fattiest and highest in cholesterol, and yet cardiovascular disease is virtually unheard of amongst them. So strange was this anomaly that, in 1974, Dr Hugh Sinclair, a medical scientist from Oxford University, went to investigate. He came back to England armed with enough seal meat, fish, crustaceans and molluscs to live off for 100 days. During that time his blood became less thick, his triglyceride (blood fat) level dropped and his HDL ('good cholesterol') level increased.[22] He had found the elixir that had protected the Inuit, a diet of foods exceptionally rich in the essential fatty acid EPA.

Thanks to the unusual diet of Sir Hugh Sinclair, since knighted for his contribution to medicine, a number of studies in the 1980s further investigated the health benefits of EPA in relation to the health of the heart and arteries. These studies fell into two categories: those that looked at the difference in cardiovascular disease between people with high or low dietary intakes of EPA; and those that gave EPA, as fish or in a capsule, to measure its effect on preventing or reversing cardiovascular disease.

In 1980 a study was carried out in Japan. Despite above average drinking and smoking, the Japanese have a record of longevity unmatched by other industrialised countries. Like the Inuit, one dietary difference is their high fish intake. An analysis of blood levels of EPA did indeed show much higher EPA in Japanese than those found in British or American populations, and especially among fish-eating, rather than farming, communities.[23] As a consequence, they may live longer and suffer less heart disease.[24]

In 1985 a study of 850 men from the Dutch town of Zutphen, followed over 20 years, found that those who ate two meals of fish a week had a lower incidence of cardiovascular disease.[25] A large-scale American MRFIT (Multiple Risk Factor Intervention Trial) study, involving 6000 men at high risk of cardiovascular disease, found that the higher the intake of Omega 3 polyunsaturated fatty acids, the lower the mortality.[26] The researchers concluded that Omega 3 fatty acids protect against cardiovascular disease. A smaller trial, published in 1994, involving 306 men and women from Edinburgh, also found a strong correlation between low levels of EPA in the blood and a high risk of cardiovascular disease.[27] These, and many other studies, indicated that there was good reason to test the effects of giving fish oil, particularly EPA, to those with cardiovascular problems.

Proven Results with Omega 3 Fish Oils

Since Dr Hugh Sinclair's discovery, dozens of proper medical trials have proved the benefit of fish oils. Here are just a few examples:

- A two-year trial for the Medical Research Council put 2000 male heart attack survivors on one of three diets. At the end of the four years, **those whose diet contained oil-rich fish or fish oil capsules had one-third fewer deaths** than those on either a low-fat or high-fibre diet.[28]

- A study on women found that **fish oil consumption lowered triglycerides, a risk factor for cardiovascular disease**.[29]

- Other studies have confirmed that **taking an EPA supplement lowers triglycerides and LDL cholesterol, thins the blood and raises HDL (good) cholesterol, as well as protecting blood fats from oxidation, all**

factors which are known to reduce cardiovascular disease.[30]

- **EPA works better than linseed oil** (which is a rich source of linolenic acid from which EPA can be made), according to a study by Sanders and Younger who compared their effects. They went on to test the effects of giving 5, 10 and 20g of EPA for three weeks. Even the lower level had positive effects, particularly on lowering triglycerides in the blood.[31]

- Dr Reg Saynor, from the Cardiothoracic Unit in Sheffield's Northern General Hospital, gave volunteers 20ml of EPA for five weeks and again found a drop in triglycerides and an increase in HDL (good) cholesterol. He continued his studies, following over 100 cardiac patients for over a year. **The supplementation of EPA resulted in virtually every person achieving normal blood triglyceride levels and much-reduced need for angina medication.**[32]

We can conclude that EPA from fish oil has five proven positive effects:

1. EPA lowers blood triglycerides (fats)
2. EPA decreases the stickiness of blood
3. EPA lowers LDL (bad) cholesterol
4. EPA raises HDL (good) cholesterol
5. EPA reduces the need for anti-angina medication

There is no drug that offers all these benefits. EPA also has a vital role to play in reducing inflammation in the artery walls and controlling insulin-resistance, a risk factor for cardiovascular disease that is discussed fully in Chapter 8.

Aspirin or EPA?

If someone has a high risk of cardiovascular disease, or indeed has had a stroke or heart attack, it is common medical practice to prescribe aspirin to thin the blood, hence reducing the risk of another blockage. Aspirin works by blocking the production of certain types of prostaglandins that increase inflammation and blood clotting. It also has many side-effects and should be used with caution by pregnant women, the elderly and children. It is also known to aggravate asthma, allergies and nasal polyps.[33] EPA doesn't have any of these side-effects and, although it thins the blood and reduces inflammation like aspirin, it also lowers blood fats and cholesterol.

Many doctors now recommend an EPA supplement (available on prescription) for those with cardiovascular risk, and sometimes prescribe it instead of or alongside other medication such as aspirin.★ Dr Rodney Foale, a Consultant Cardiologist at St Mary's Hospital, London, recommends fish oil supplements to anyone with a risk of cardiovascular disease who does not eat oily fish two to three times a week.

It may also be useful for those with diabetes, as one of the disease's more serious side-effects is poor circulation caused by arterial disease. In a study on 20 patients with diabetes, the inclusion of fish oil, rich in EPA, in their diet significantly improved circulation in six weeks, compared to those taking olive oil.[34]

Of course, prevention is better than cure, and, like the Inuit, you may choose to add EPA to your diet to minimise your risk of cardiovascular disease.

★One word of caution: both fish oil and aspirin thin the blood. The combined use of large amounts of both could cause a potentially harmful condition in which the blood fails to clot, leading to prolonged bleeding times in the case of injury. Therefore it may be prudent not to combine on-going aspirin and high-dose fish oil unless recommended to do so by your doctor.[35]

The Role of Omega 6 Oils

While the main focus of attention has been on the Omega 3 family of essential fats, mainly found in fish oils, there are also proven benefits from taking the other type of essential fats, the Omega 6 family. These are found in cold-pressed sunflower, sesame and walnut oils; but the most active form, known as gamma-linolenic acid (GLA), comes from evening primrose oil and borage oil (sometimes called starflower oil). Professor Renaud, of the French National Institute for Health and Medical Research in Lyons, studied the population of Crete, where the incidence of cardiovascular disease is among the lowest in the world.[36] He found that they had 68 per cent more GLA in their blood than average. GLA, like EPA, is a natural anti-coagulant and anti-inflammatory agent which prevents the formation of blood clots and is well worth including in your diet.

······································

CHAPTER 7

LIPOPROTEIN (A) – THE VITAMIN C CONNECTION

Recent discoveries in environmental science, evolution and genetics are beginning to unravel the mystery of how we, as a species, have evolved. It now appears that many diseases we label as bad may have actually developed to protect us. When your nose blocks up on exposure to a pollutant, or when the cells in a smoker's lungs change their form after repeated exposure to poisons in a cigarette, the body is trying to adapt to new conditions. It is this very ability to adapt that keeps us alive in an ever-changing world.

At the age of 92, Dr Linus Pauling, a scientific genius with two Nobel Prizes to his name, proposed that the development of cardiovascular disease, the number one killer in the Western world, may have prevented our extinction. His paper, 'A Unified Theory of Human Cardiovascular Disease', co-authored by Dr Matthias Rath, has attracted considerable interest among leading cardiologists.[37] If proved right, this theory will not only largely solve the riddle of the origin of heart disease, but may lead to its abolition as a cause of human death. The solution? Vitamin C.

THE VITAMIN C STORY

All animals, except guinea pigs, fruit-eating bats, the red-vented bulbul bird and primates, make vitamin C in their bodies. The amount varies from creature to creature but is usually in the human equivalent of between 1000 and 20,000mg per day. Most people in the Western world currently consume below 100mg. About 40 million years ago our ancestors lost this ability to synthesise vitamin C from glucose; as a result, we now depend entirely on dietary sources.

This genetic mutation probably occurred because we had sufficient supplies in our diet. Indeed, our ancestors' diet, being rich in fruits and other plant material, could easily have provided several grams per day. When our ancestors left tropical regions, however, to settle in other parts of the world (especially during the Ice Age, when vegetation was very scarce), they would have been at high risk of developing scurvy (vitamin C deficiency).

Scurvy is a fatal disease. It is characterised by a breakdown of the connective tissue that holds us together. Ascorbate (vitamin C) is essential in the production of collagen and elastin, which bind our skin, membranes and cells. The first sign of scurvy is vascular bleeding, as blood vessels start to leak – their membranes are under more pressure than any others in the body, because of the force of blood pumping through them. Blood loss from scurvy decimated ships' crews in the earlier part of this century. It is quite conceivable that death from scurvy could have decimated the human species, especially during the thousands of years of Ice Ages.

Nature on the Defensive

So how did we survive? According to Pauling and Rath, we may have developed the ability to deposit lipids (fats) along the artery walls to protect them from deteriorating and bleeding, in order to increase our chances of surviving during ascorbate–deficient times.[38] Another group of proteins that normally accumulate at injury sites to effect repair are fibrinogen and apoprotein. Lipids and apoprotein combine to produce lipoprotein (a) which, in excess, is now thought to be a good predictor of impending cardiovascular disease.

Lipoprotein (a) can repair damaged or leaky blood vessels, but it also increases the risk of heart disease by building up deposits on artery walls.[39] Research is now strongly suggesting that the development of lipoprotein (a) was a genetic response to the threat of extinction due to leaky blood vessels. Could this have been nature's way of protecting us from life-threatening scurvy? The estimated period of the development of lipoprotein (a) in monkeys coincides with the time at which primates are thought to have lost the ability to produce vitamin C.

So, how well does the theory of vitamin C deficiency as a root cause for cardiovascular disease fit the facts? A lack of vitamin C raises blood levels of cholesterol, triglycerides, the 'bad' LDLs, apoprotein (a) and lipoprotein (a), and lowers the beneficial HDLs. Conversely, increasing vitamin C intake lowers high cholesterol, triglycerides, LDL or lipoprotein (a) levels and raises HDLs. The chance of all these effects being unconnected was too small – Pauling, Rath and their colleagues wanted to investigate further.

One theory is that for our ancestors, during the summer months when vitamin C intake was sufficient, the increased HDL production would remove excess cholesterol. Vitamin C also inhibits excessive cholesterol production and stimulates a key enzyme for converting cholesterol to bile (necessary for digestion). All this would lead to a decrease in unnecessary atherosclerotic deposits. In one study it was shown that 500mg of vitamin C a day can lead to a reduction in atherosclerotic deposits within two to six months. 'This concept also explains why heart attack and stroke occur today with a much higher frequency in winter than during spring and summer, the seasons with increased ascorbate intake,' says Pauling.

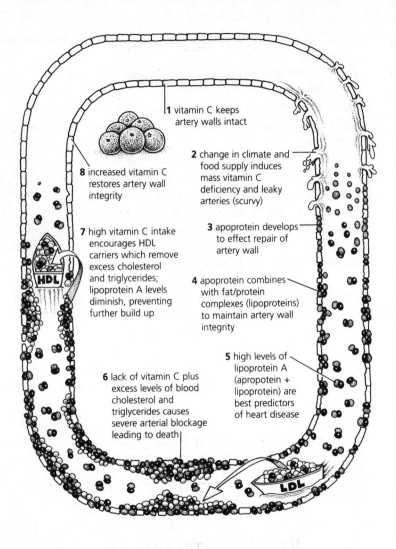

1 vitamin C keeps artery walls intact

2 change in climate and food supply induces mass vitamin C deficiency and leaky arteries (scurvy)

3 apoprotein develops to effect repair of artery wall

4 apoprotein combines with fat/protein complexes (lipoproteins) to maintain artery wall integrity

5 high levels of lipoprotein A (apropotein + lipoprotein) are best predictors of heart disease

6 lack of vitamin C plus excess levels of blood cholesterol and triglycerides causes severe arterial blockage leading to death

7 high vitamin C intake encourages HDL carriers which remove excess cholesterol and triglycerides; lipoprotein A levels diminish, preventing further build up

8 increased vitamin C restores artery wall integrity

HDL

LDL

Fig 7 – How Vitamin C is Linked to the Cause and Cure of Arterial Disease

GENETIC EVIDENCE

There is strong evidence that some people have a genetic tendency to develop high cholesterol or high triglycerides or both. According to Pauling's theory, a lack of vitamin C unmasks this tendency, which developed to protect our arteries from scurvy.

Two other genetically based cardiovascular diseases are diabetic angiopathy and homocysteinuria. In diabetes, the very high levels of glucose in the blood interfere with vitamin C intake and speed up degeneration of the arteries. Taking a vitamin C supplement not only helps to prevent these problems by increasing its concentration in artery walls but also improves blood glucose and insulin balance.

Homocysteinuria is another genetic disorder (discussed in detail in Chapter 9), in which the sufferer accumulates an excess of toxic homocysteine. Such an excess causes damage throughout the cardiovascular system – 60 per cent of patients show clinical signs before the age of 40. Once again, vitamin C supplementation can prevent these problems, and other complications of the disease, by helping people to metabolise homocysteine properly.

Low, Medium and High Risk Lipoprotein (a) Levels

Low	Medium	High
10mg/dl	20mg/dl	30mg/dl

REVERSING ATHEROSCLEROSIS

Of course, the proof of any theory lies in whether or not it works. Treatment for atherosclerosis (build-up of deposits on artery walls) involves taking vitamin C and the amino acid lysine, which together help to prevent lipoprotein (a) from binding to arterial walls, and also helps to remove arterial deposits, thereby reversing atherosclerosis.[40] No clinical trials to test this theory have yet been completed, but an increasing number of success stories are being reported. In fact, since the publication of Pauling and Rath's theories, no less than 1100 research papers have made reference to lipoprotein (a). One, from the University of Arkansas for Medical Sciences, reported a 35 per cent decrease in lipoprotein (a) after 26 weeks on niacin[41] which proves even more effective in combination with vitamin C and lysine.

So far, the anecdotal evidence is very encouraging. One such case involves a leading US biochemist who had had three coronary bypass operations, numerous complications, and angina (heart pain) at the slightest exertion. He took many daily medications, including beta-blockers and aspirin. To this medication his cardiologist, who confirmed that a fourth coronary bypass operation was not possible, advised him to add 6g of ascorbic acid (vitamin C), 60mg of Co-Q10, a multivitamin tablet with minerals, additional vitamins A, E and B complex, lecithin and niacin (B3). Linus Pauling recommended he continue the ascorbic acid and add 5g of lysine daily.

The biochemist started with 1g of lysine in May 1991, and increased the daily dose to 5g by mid-June. By mid-July he could walk 3km (2 miles) and do gardening work without angina pain and wrote: 'The effect of the lysine borders on the miraculous.' He attributes his newfound well-being to the addition of lysine and vitamins to his other medications. His wife and friends have all commented on his renewed vigour.

Likewise, a patient of mine, who had had three strokes and had suffered from high blood pressure for ten years, came to me suffering from angina due to a blocked coronary artery. Even a brisk walk gave him extreme chest pain. He took 5g of vitamin C and 3g of lysine, plus 600iu of vitamin E and 30mg of Co-Q 10. Five months later, having stopped taking two drugs for high blood pressure, his blood pressure was normal and he could raise his exercising pulse rate to 180 beats per minute before experiencing any pain.

Another patient who had suffered a major heart attack was left unable to walk up any incline due to severe angina. Within three months on vitamin C and lysine he was able to walk up hills again. Yet another man who believes Linus Pauling brought him back from the brink of death is David Holmes. Writing in the journal, *Holistic Health*,[42] he tells his story: 'At the age of 48 I had a sudden and quite severe heart attack with no prior warning symptoms.' After that he devised an excellent nutritional prevention strategy:

All went very well for about seventeen years. But in August 1993 I began to suffer from angina pains when making very short walks of some 20 yards. My blood tests showed that my blood chemistry was normal in most respects: low in cholesterol, high in HDL. My blood analysis also showed something else. It showed a dangerously high lipoprotein (a). I began taking 1g L–lysine and 1g vitamin C in three separate doses thrice daily. Over three weeks I increased these amounts up to a total of 6g lysine and 6g vitamin C. Other supplements I added were Omega 3 fatty acids and magnesium. On this new regime my angina became less and less frequent and my exercise tolerance increased as the days went by. Subsequent blood tests showed a dramatic fall in both lipoprotein (a) and apolipoprotein A2 (another potential harmful lipoprotein). Having reduced both the lipoprotein (a) and apolipoprotein A2 to normal, the angina became much less frequent so that some three months after beginning I was able to go to the Maritime Alps and walk three to six miles per day up and down the mountains without pain for three weeks at Christmas time. Finally, I was able to stop the beta-blocker Atenolol and Diltiazem completely.

A RADICAL RETHINK ON HEART DISEASE

Pauling and Rath's theory on the cause and treatment of heart disease certainly fits the facts at hand but will inevitably need to be thoroughly tested, in predicting, treating and preventing cardiovascular disease, before it will receive wide acceptance. If proved right, however, it will necessitate a radical rethink by all those scientists who have pursued other models such as the cholesterol theory. According to scientist Max Planck, 'An important innovation rarely makes its way by gradually winning over and converting its opponents. What does happen is that its opponents gradually die out and that the growing generation is familiar with the idea from the beginning.' The vitamin C theory may be one such idea.

Pauling, who died in 1994 at the age of 93, was certainly convinced that, 'Cardiovascular disease is the direct consequence of the inability of man to synthesise ascorbate in combination with insufficient intake of ascorbate in the modern diet.' If vitamin C deficiency does prove to be a major cause of human cardiovascular disease, then vitamin C supplementation is destined to become the universal treatment for this disease. He recommends somewhere between 5 and 20g per day, together with the amino acid l-lysine. The available epidemiological and clinical evidence is reasonably convincing. In Dr Linus Pauling's words, 'Further clinical confirmation of this theory should lead to the abolition of cardiovascular disease as a cause of human mortality for the present generation and future generations of mankind.'

CHAPTER 8

INSULIN-RESISTANCE – THE SUGAR FACTOR

In both the US and the UK, calorie intake and the consumption of fat throughout the population are going down, yet rates of obesity are going up! So much for excess fat or calories being the cause of weight gain. This anomaly is, however, explained by our ever-decreasing levels of exercise and a highly significant, yet little known risk factor for cardiovascular disease now thought to affect a quarter of the population – insulin-resistance. Because of this syndrome, first identified by Gerald Reaven, Professor of Medicine at Stanford University Medical School, as many as one in four people respond abnormally to eating carbohydrates (sugar, grains, fruit, etc) by over-producing insulin.[43] The job of this hormone is to transport glucose (the end product of the digestion of carbohydrate) from the blood to the cells in the body. The trouble is, some people become resistant to insulin; in effect, the insulin doesn't work so the body keeps producing more to achieve its aim of lowering the blood glucose levels. Consequently, blood glucose and insulin levels tend to stay higher for longer after a meal containing carbohydrate. But what's all this got to do with heart disease?

INSULIN-RESISTANCE AND YOUR HEART

In the same way as smoking introduces oxidants into the body which damage the arteries, so too does excess blood glucose.

The process is called glycation and it is now recognised as a leading cause of arterial damage in those with adult-onset diabetes, in which a person's resistance to insulin becomes so great that they can no longer lower their blood glucose levels. Their blood sugar levels therefore stay too high (the condition known as diabetes) and their body cells fail to get their delivery of glucose, leading to exhaustion.

It is glycation, or sugar coating, that causes the damage to eyes, kidneys and nerves in those with diabetes. This excess glucose also damages cholesterol and essential fats, increasing the 'bad' LDL cholesterol and triglycerides (partly due to insulin's effects on the liver). Having too much insulin in the blood also inflames the arteries and raises blood pressure. All this adds up to an increased risk of cardiovascular disease as a result of:

- Hypertension (50 per cent of high blood pressure patients are insulin-resistant)
- Poor cholesterol status and elevated triglycerides
- Increased fibrinogen levels
- Elevated uric acid (associated with gout)

Probably the major way in which having too much insulin, known as hyperinsulinemia, increases the risk of cardiovascular disease is by causing the body to turn essential fats into the wrong kind of prostaglandins (discussed in Chapter 6) which, in turn, influence hormone balance. While the prostaglandins made from Omega 3 oils, rich in fish, are good for the arteries, the prostaglandins made from Omega 6 oils can be good or bad. Excess insulin switches the body's metabolism of Omega 6 to produce a prostaglandin called PGE2 which causes inflammation in the arteries and atherosclerosis. PGE2s are also made in the body directly from meat and dairy produce, which may be one of the main reasons why a high consumption of these foods is associated with an increased risk of cardiovascular disease.

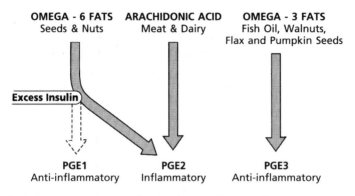

Fig 8 – How Excess Insulin Leads to Inflammation

Virtually everyone with diabetes or blood sugar problems, but also one in four ordinary people, have this kind of altered metabolism[44] and, as a result, are at risk of cardiovascular disease, especially if they eat a high carbohydrate diet of bread, pasta, cereals and fruit. Of course, this is exactly the diet we are told is good for us! And so it is, provided you don't have insulin–resistance. Even worse for those with this altered metabolism is a diet of refined foods, sugar, stimulants such as tea and coffee, and a stressful lifestyle. In fact, having too much insulin also alters the balance of adrenal hormones in the body, encouraging stressful reactions.

By now you may be asking two questions: do I have insulin–resistance, and if so, what on earth should I be eating? The first question can be answered by completing the Insulin-Resistance Questionnaire (see page 48), devised by Antony Haynes, an expert in nutrition and cardiovascular health. The answer to the second question depends on the answer to the first. We now know that the ideal diet for a person with insulin–resistance is different from the ideal diet for someone without this tendency. What is more, the right kind of diet can actually normalise your metabolism and substantially reduce your risk of a heart attack.

Are you insulin-resistant?

According to Dr Barry Sears, author of the book *Enter The Zone*[45] which spells out a dietary strategy to reset your metabolism, lose weight, decrease cardiovascular risk and maximise performance by stabilising your blood sugar and insulin levels, 'If you're fat and you're shaped like an apple, you're hyperinsulinemic, and you don't need a medical test to tell you. It is also quite possible to be lean and have elevated insulin levels.' The Insulin-Resistance Questionnaire will give you a better idea of the likelihood of this. If your risk is high I definitely recommend that you work with a nutrition consultant or well-informed doctor to run tests and devise a special dietary regime which can correct your metabolism in as little as three months.

Insulin-Resistance Questionnaire

Section 1: Case History
- Do you have a family history of diabetes? **Yes / No**
- Do you get indigestion after meals? **Yes / No**
- Do you get sleepy after meals? **Yes / No**
- Do you have high fat stores, although not obese? **Yes / No**
- Do you get oedema (water retention)? **Yes / No**
- Do you take regular anaerobic exercise? **Yes / No**
- Do you have addictions, especially to carbohydrates or chocolate? **Yes / No**
- Do you take the birth control pill? **Yes / No**
- Are you above 60 years of age? **Yes / No**
- Do you drink four or more cups of caffeinated drinks daily? **Yes / No**
- Do you sweat a lot or get excessively thirsty? **Yes / No**
- Do you get dizzy or irritable if you don't eat often? **Yes / No**
- Do you have increased fat stores in spite of exercise and low-calorie diet but still have approximately normal weight for your height? **Yes / No**

- Are you more than 7kg (14 lb) over your ideal weight? **Yes / No**
- Are you tired all the time? **Yes / No**
- Do you get cravings for something sweet after meals? **Yes / No**
- Do you have a sedentary lifestyle? **Yes / No**

Total Answers 'Yes' =

Section 2: Examination and Tests

- Do you have elevated fasting triglycerides? **Yes / No**
- Do you have elevated cholesterol? **Yes / No**
- Do you have low HDL levels? **Yes / No**
- Do you have elevated LDL levels? **Yes / No**
- Do you have elevated blood pressure? **Yes / No**
- Do you have elevated levels of glycosylated haemoglobin (HgBA1C)? **Yes / No**
- Do you have elevated two-hour post-prandial insulin? **Yes / No**
- Do you have elevated fasting glucose levels? **Yes / No**
- Do you have elevated two-hour post-prandial glucose? **Yes / No**
- Do you have low DHEA(S) levels? **Yes / No**
- Do you have postural hypotension? **Yes / No**
  (*i.e. your blood pressure drops upon standing*)
- Do you have an increased waist-to-hip ratio and are you apple-shaped? **Yes / No**

Total Answers 'Yes' =

Section 1: If you have answered 'Yes' to question 1 then you should seek the advice of a nutritionist or doctor trained in this area, as insulin-resistance is more likely in those with first-degree relatives.

Yes Answers Category

8–5	*Category One – Stable Blood Sugar Levels*
5–10	*Category Two – Minor Imbalances*
11–17	*Category Three – Marked Imbalances*

Section 2:
Yes Answers Category

0	*Category One – Stable Blood Sugar Levels likely*
1–3	*Potential for Category Three – further investigation required.*
4–12	*It is recommended that you see a doctor trained in this area, as well as seeking appropriate nutritional support.*

IS HEART DISEASE AN INFLAMMATORY CONDITION?

For someone with insulin-resistance, the priority is to calm down the inflammation caused by PGE2 and stabilise the blood sugar level. One way to do this is to take an aspirin. Aspirin reduces the production of PGE2. However it also reduces the production of the beneficial anti–inflammatory prostaglandins, but not so quickly. The net result is a mild anti–inflammatory effect. This, coupled with the fact that aspirin thins the blood, is probably why it is associated with a slight reduction in heart attack risk.

Indeed, so significant is the inflammation that occurs in damaged arteries that the degree of inflammation is now being used to predict risk. A test has recently been developed to measure the presence of a substance called C-reactive protein. This substance reflects the degree of inflammation, and can predict heart disease risk many years before standard diagnostic tests find clogged arteries. Having a high level of C-reactive protein triples a person's risk for heart disease. What's more, according to research carried out at Emory University in Atlanta, aspirin only works if there is arterial inflammation. A much more sophisticated way to reduce inflammation, without a downside, is to change what you are eating.

EATING YOUR WAY OUT OF INSULIN-RESISTANCE

Basically, there are three key elements to eating your way out of insulin-resistance. (**Please note**: these guidelines are specifically for those with insulin-resistance and do not constitute an ideal diet for those with stable blood sugar levels.)

1. Change the balance of protein and carbohydrate in each meal.

While a high-carbohydrate meal leads to high blood glucose and insulin levels, eating more protein with your carbohydrate has the effect of stabilising glucose and insulin levels. So too does avoiding sugar and refined carbohydrates and only eating whole foods containing complex carbohydrates.

2. Eat more fish and fish oils, and less meat and dairy produce.

The goal here is to decrease the formation of PGE2s by limiting red meat and dairy produce and increasing your intake of Omega 3 oils, either by eating carnivorous fish (salmon, tuna, herring, mackerel, etc) three times a week, or by taking an EPA fish oil supplement.

3. Increase your intake of antioxidants.

These are vital for everyone but especially so for those with insulin-resistance. While antioxidants such as vitamin E protect essential fats in the body, they also protect the arteries from oxidant damage caused by excess glucose (glycation). Lipoic acid (another antioxidant), available as a supplement, also regenerates both vitamin C and vitamin E.

Finally, it's also important to take regular aerobic exercise such as brisk walking, jogging, cycling, swimming or exercise classes. This is because aerobic exercise is known to increase the body's sensitivity to insulin – so it's all the more important for those with insulin-resistance.

BALANCING PROTEIN AND CARBOHYDRATE

Hippocrates was dead right when he said 'let food be your medicine and medicine your food' – we now know that changing the balance of fat, protein and carbohydrate in our diet can have significant consequences for our health. While the general guidelines for healthy eating recommend a high complex carbohydrate diet (60–70 per cent of calories) and modest protein (15–20 per cent), for those with insulin-resistance this otherwise healthy diet can make matters worse, not better. The reason for this is that eating carbohydrates stimulates insulin production, while protein stimulates a hormone called glucagon which stabilises insulin levels and helps the body use fats for energy. Therefore, the greater the degree of insulin-resistance, the greater the need to eat more protein in relation to carbohydrate in each meal. This is because, to quote a recent article in the *American Journal of Clinical Nutrition*, 'Protein metabolism is impaired in insulin resistance and the degree to which protein metabolism is related to insulin levels is more important than was previously thought.'[46]

For those in Category 2 and 3 from the Insulin-Resistance Questionnaire, the amount of protein consumed needs to go up to between 20 and 40 per cent of calories, but only for a short time, perhaps three months maximum (because long-term over-consumption of protein has a downside too). In practical terms, this means that if you eat rice, pasta, bread or potatoes you should cut down the portion size and have a substantial portion of a protein-rich food as well.

Examples of such combinations are fish and rice; chicken or soya sausages with potatoes; a tuna fish sandwich; tofu and vegetable steam-fry; pasta with tofu or tuna. One high-quality protein grain is quinoa, a staple food in South America. It is

20 per cent protein, the rest being mainly carbohydrate. So, for a vegan, quinoa, tofu and vegetables would be an excellent way to eat a healthy meal containing around 30 per cent protein. The ideal balance is two parts carbohydrate to one part protein. As far as snacks are concerned, this would also mean not eating fruit on its own; instead you would eat fruit with high-protein nuts such as almonds. Apples are the best fruit as they release their sugar content slowly.

According to nutritionist Antony Haynes:

Depending on the severity of the imbalances, most people need to follow such a corrective diet for a minimum of two months before a gradual return to a higher carbohydrate diet may become possible without adverse effects. However, for some people there will be a need to consume protein of a high class (e.g. animal protein, quinoa or soy products) for longer than this. Vegans may be at particular risk of exacerbating any existing insulin resistance or potential for it due to their reduced high class protein intake, unless they consume soy products regularly.

MICRONUTRIENTS AND INSULIN-RESISTANCE

Micronutrients (vitamins, minerals, etc) also play a significant role in controlling insulin, glucose and oxidation and hence cardiovascular health. Taking a chromium supplement, for example, raises HDL cholesterol, presumably because it helps to stabilise blood sugar levels. The judicious use of vitamins and minerals, together with the right balance of protein and carbohydrate, is the safest and most effective way to correct insulin–resistance and restore the body's normal metabolism. Here is a guide to the most important nutrients showing the recommended dosage range and their effects. Depending on your status from the questionnaire these micronutrients may be important for you:

Using Micronutrients to Improve Cardiovascular Health

Nutrient	Dosage range	Effect
GLA	100–200 mg	Both anti-inflammatory and
EPA	400–800 mg	improve insulin function
L-carnitine	400–2000 mg	Helps metabolise fats
Chromium	50–300 mcg	Stabilises glucose levels
Magnesium	200–600 mg	Improves insulin function
Zinc	15–25 mg	Improves insulin function
N-acetylcysteine	50–2000 mg	Antioxidant
Co-Q10	10–200 mg	Antioxidant
Lipoic acid	10–500 mg	Antioxidant and anti-glycation
Vitamin E	100–1000 mg	Antioxidant and anti-glycation

The highest dosages are only applicable to those in category 3, under the guidance of a nutrition consultant or doctor.

DIFFERENT COURSES FOR DIFFERENT HORSES

Not all the above micronutrients may be advisable or necessary for you. Generally speaking, if you have a marked imbalance in glucose and insulin (Category 3) it is highly advisable to see a nutrition consultant who can design a corrective diet and supplement programme specifically for you. This will often start with high levels of antioxidants and no supplementation of essential fats such as EPA. This is because these essential fats can easily be damaged or oxidised so the first step is to improve your body's antioxidant status and ability to protect essential fats. Once this is achieved, taking an EPA supplement is very beneficial and it is better to follow the guidelines for the Category 2 diet below. If you scored low on the Insulin-Resistance Questionnaire, then the Category 1 Diet is most appropriate for you. Part 5 of this book explains what this means in terms of what to eat. At present, you only need to understand the basic principles.

Dietary Action Plans

Category 1: Stable Blood Sugar Levels
- High unrefined carbohydrate   60–70 per cent
- Modest protein   15–20 per cent
- Low fat with adequate: 10–20 per cent
  B vitamins, chromium, zinc
  magnesium and antioxidants

Category 2: Minor Imbalances
- Modest unrefined carbohydrate   45–60 per cent
- Increased protein   20–25 per cent
- Modest fat with additional:
  Omega 3 EPA (low saturated fat)
  and monounsaturates, magnesium,
  chromium, zinc and B vitamins

Category 3: Marked Imbalances
- Management of carbohydrate   40–50 per cent
  to lower oxidative stress
- More protein and glycogenic   30–40 per cent
  (energy-giving) amino acids:
  e.g. supplemental glutamine,
  leucine, isoleucine, valine
- High dose mitochondrial
  antioxidant support:
  vitamin E, lipoic
  acid, glutathione, L-carnitine,
  co-Enzyme Q10, magnesium,
  chromium, zinc

CHAPTER 9

HOMOCYSTEINE – THE HEART ATTACKER

Once arteries become damaged there's a whole sequence of events that leads to the development of plaque, thickening and the eventual risk of a total blockage. But what causes the damage in the first place? We know that a lack of vitamin C fundamentally weakens the artery wall, making it more prone to damage. Also, a high intake of oxidants (for example, from smoking or eating fried foods) may lead to increasing arterial damage, especially if the person is deficient in antioxidants such as vitamin C and E. But there is another, more insidious factor produced by the body that is at least as dangerous as having high cholesterol – homocysteine.

The homocysteine theory was first proposed by Dr Kilmer McCully, a pathologist at the VA Medical Center in Providence, Rhode Island, USA, in 1969. He had been studying a rare genetic disorder called homocysteinuria. Children born with this condition lack certain enzymes required to turn the toxic substance homocysteine into harmless cystanthionine. Unless they are diagnosed and treated, these children often die of heart attacks and strokes before reaching adulthood, despite having completely normal cholesterol levels.

Homocysteine is made from protein in the diet. The amino acid methionine is converted into homocysteine in the body and, provided you have enough vitamin B6, B12 and folic

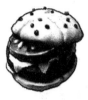

1 Protein rich foods contain an amino acid, methionine, that converts to homocysteine

2 Excess levels of homocysteine damages the lining of arteries

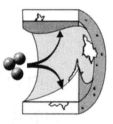

3 Cholesterol builds up inside the scarred arteries, which can lead to fatal blockages

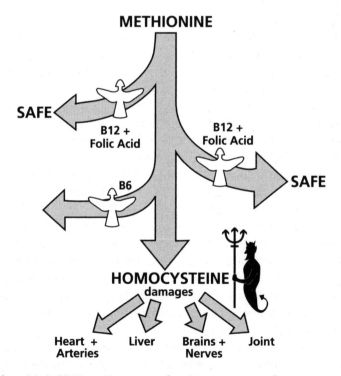

METHIONINE

SAFE

B12 + Folic Acid

B12 + Folic Acid

SAFE

B6

HOMOCYSTEINE damages

Heart + Arteries

Liver

Brains + Nerves

Joint

Fig – 9A & 9B How Homocysteine Damages Arteries

acid, the body will convert it into cystanthionine. We now know that homocysteine is very toxic and can cause the initial damage to the artery wall that starts the whole process of cardiovascular disease.

Although the genetic disease homocysteinuria is rare, McCully wondered what percentage of people produced small excesses of homocysteine which, over many years, might increase their risk. He also wondered to what extent homocysteine excess was limited to those with a genetic predisposition or could occur in anyone lacking vitamin B6, B12 or folic acid, deficiencies of which are extremely common. As his investigation unfolded he found that smoking and inactivity tended to raise homocysteine levels and that those with a family history of heart disease often shared a minor flaw in one of the genes governing homocysteine metabolism.

Homocysteine levels rise with age; women have, on average, 20 per cent lower levels than men, until the menopause. Then levels between the sexes are more or less equal. All these findings fitted perfectly with the incidence of heart attacks occurring more often in smoking, sedentary men, and then rising in women after the menopause. It was also well known that injecting animals with homocysteine produced arterial plaque.

PROVING THE HOMOCYSTEINE THEORY

It wasn't until the nineties that the evidence for the homocysteine theory started to become very convincing.[47] In 1992 a study of 14,000 male doctors found that those who had the top 5 per cent of homocysteine levels had three times the heart attack risk of those who had the bottom 5 per cent. This was confirmed by the Massachusetts-based Framingham Heart Study in 1995 which found that having more than 11.4 micromoles per litre of homocysteine in the blood increased the risk.[48] Another study at the University of Washington found that having high homocysteine levels doubled the risk of heart attack in young women.

The real clincher was a study carried out by the European Concerted Action Group, a consortium of doctors and researchers from 19 medical centres in nine European countries.[49] Having studied 750 people under the age of 60 with atherosclerosis, compared to 800 people without such cardiovascular disease, they found that having a high level of homocysteine in the blood was as great a risk factor as smoking or having a high blood cholesterol level. Those in the top fifth of homocysteine levels had double the risk of cardiovascular disease. In other words, 20 per cent of the people tested had double the risk of cardiovascular disease because of high homocysteine levels.

They also found that those taking vitamin supplements reduced their risk to a third of those not taking supplements. When they compared blood levels of vitamin B6, B12 and folic acid they found that there was a direct relationship between increasing homocysteine levels and decreasing levels of folic acid and vitamin B6, with vitamin B6 being the strongest association. B12 status didn't correlate with homocysteine levels.

CAN VITAMIN B6 AND FOLIC ACID PREVENT HEART DISEASE?

There is no doubt that homocysteine has a role to play in cardiovascular disease. Those most at risk are high protein (meat) eaters with a poor intake of vitamin B6, B12 and folic acid. While meat is considered a reasonable source of vitamin B6, one survey found that you needed to eat at least five hamburgers a day to achieve the basic RDA of vitamin B6 which is 2mg. A hamburger diet is therefore high in protein, high in saturated fat and cholesterol and clearly deficient in both vitamin B6 and folic acid. Better foods for B6 and folic acid are green leafy vegetables, nuts, whole grains, wheatgerm, fish and free-range chicken.

However, researchers are recommending higher levels of these vitamins than can easily be gained from diet alone, namely at least 10 to 50mg of vitamin B6 and 400 to 1000mcg of folic acid, plus 10mcg of B12. As *Newsweek* reported in August 1997, 'It may turn out that we can achieve more with nickel-and-dime vitamin supplements than with drugs that cost hundreds of times more.'

CHAPTER 10

MAGNESIUM AND THE HEART ATTACK MYSTERY

Maria, an elderly lady, had angina. Although there was evidence of atherosclerosis in her coronary arteries this didn't fully explain her angina attacks, which didn't fit the usual pattern of pain on exertion or after eating a large or high-fat meal. Her doctors advised a coronary bypass operation, to bypass partially blocked arteries. As they were performing the operation they witnessed something unusual and life-threatening. One of her coronary arteries went into complete spasm, becoming stiff and hard. They were witnessing a coronary artery spasm, now known to occur when there is severe magnesium deficiency. This is the likely explanation for a small number of heart attack victims who, on autopsy, are not found to have complete arterial blockage.

This story explains the known connection between having a low level of magnesium and a high risk of heart disease. In fact, heart attack victims tend to have 30 per cent less magnesium and a higher calcium level than normal.[50,51] Cardiovascular risk is also higher in parts of the world where either the dietary intake of magnesium or the level of magnesium in the water is low. The risk of heart disease is lower in hard water areas, where the water provides more calcium and magnesium. Modern diets are deficient in magnesium, which is high in vegetables, nuts, seeds and wholefoods, and low in refined foods, meat and dairy produce. The average diet only provides 200mg a day (compared to the RDA of 300mg or the optimal intake of 500mg). Perhaps our decreasing levels of magnesium, which is involved in over 300 essential chemical processes in the body, is one reason why we are witnessing an epidemic of heart disease.

RELAX WITH MAGNESIUM

One of the main roles of magnesium, together with calcium, is to control the contraction and relaxation of muscles. Both calcium and magnesium atoms can hold an electrical charge. Their balance inside and outside a muscle cell determines whether the muscle cell will contract or relax.

Since arteries contain a layer of muscle, Professors Burton and Bella Altura, a husband and wife team from the State University of New York's Health Science Center, wondered whether a deficiency in magnesium could cause an artery to spasm, thus reducing or cutting off blood supply. Their research,[52] which spanned three decades, proved conclusively that removing magnesium from the environment of blood vessels made them go into spasm, potentially reducing the diameter of an artery to one-third of its normal size, as shown below.

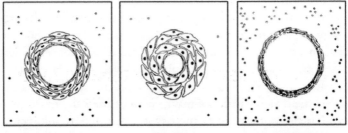

Normal Calcium
and Magnesium

Normal Calcium
and low
Magnesium

Normal Calcium
and high
Magnesium

Fig 10 – How Magnesium Relaxes Arteries

If a person's arteries were already narrowed due to athero-sclerosis, such a level of magnesium reduction could initiate a heart attack or stroke. Their research also added a new, inexpensive and harmless therapy for cardiovascular disease – the essential mineral magnesium.

Increasing magnesium intake, especially for those with borderline deficiency, immediately lowers blood pressure. As long ago as 1977, researchers from Georgetown University demonstrated an 11 per cent decrease in blood pressure by giving magnesium to people with hypertension.[53] Since then, the relaxing effects on the arteries of magnesium, which also helps reduce anxiety and insomnia, has been well established by numerous research groups. What's more, people with high blood pressure frequently show lower levels of magnesium than those with normal blood pressure.

So, optimal magnesium intake not only protects us from high blood pressure, for those at cardiovascular risk it also reduces the danger of a heart attack. Giving magnesium, usually by injection, during a heart attack also helps stabilise the heart and dramatically reduces the risk of death.

While much of the research into magnesium's protective effects has focussed on its relaxing role in arteries, there is growing evidence that magnesium can also reduce cholesterol and triglyceride levels.[54] Indeed, having a low level of magnesium is as great a risk for cardiovascular disease as having a high cholesterol level.

ARE YOU GETTING ENOUGH MAGNESIUM?

The worst diet, from the point of view of both heart disease and low magnesium, is high in meat, milk, refined foods, sugar and saturated fat. Not only is such a diet deficient in magnesium, it's also high in calcium. The body needs the right balance of these two 'push-me-pull-you' minerals, which control both nerve and muscle function. Too much calcium in relation to magnesium can cause muscle cramping, irregular heartbeat, high blood pressure, nervousness, irritability and insomnia.

Alternatively, eating a diet rich in vegetables, fruit, nuts and seeds provides more than enough magnesium and calcium. This is how our ancestors got their calcium. After all, they weren't milking buffaloes! The best seeds are pumpkin, followed by sunflower and sesame, while the best nuts are almonds and cashews. Half a cup of pumpkin seeds provides 370mg of magnesium (the ideal daily intake being between 300 and 500mg). Another great food for magnesium is wheatgerm. A spoonful of wheatgerm and ground pumpkin seeds added to your morning cereal ensures added protection against heart disease.

....

CHAPTER 11

ACQUIRED OR INHERITED?

Cardiovascular disease often runs in families – a factor which led to the debate on whether we inherit it from our parents or acquire it through diet and lifestyle habits. The answer is both. In previous chapters we saw how too much cholesterol, triglycerides, homocysteine and lipoprotein all predict an increased risk of cardiovascular disease. The tendency to over-produce these substances appears to be partly inherited, yet your diet can not only prevent these risk factors ever emerging, but also reverse the risk once it has developed. This means that, even if you have a family history of cardiovascular disease, you don't have to suffer. In any case, family histories of disease often turn out to have nothing to do with inheriting genetic predispositions as such. Rather, they occur due to inheriting certain lifestyle and dietary habits that put you at risk. In both cases the good news is that you *can* do something about it. This is especially encouraging, since it is a lot easier to improve your diet than change your genes. And the earlier you start, the better.

DOES HEART DISEASE START IN THE WOMB?

Thanks to the extraordinary work of Professor Barker and colleagues at the Environmental Epidemiology Unit at Southampton University, we now know that cardiovascular disease can be 'programmed' during foetal development, depending on the nutrition a foetus receives from its mother during pregnancy.

The researchers found that those born with a low birth weight had a high risk of hypertension, diabetes and cardio-vascular disease later in life. Other surveys found double the risk of cardiovascular disease or diabetes in infants who were thin at birth or short in terms of body length.

To investigate this new risk factor more fully, Professor Barker collaborated with researchers from Helsinki University Central Hospital in Finland in a remarkable study of 3302 men born in the hospital between 1924 and 1933.[55] Since Finland has one of the highest cardiovascular disease rates in the world and an excellent system for recording details at birth, here was a unique opportunity to put the 'foetal pro-gramming' theory to the test. They tracked down each of these 3302 men to determine whether they were alive, and, if so, the state of their health, and if not, their cause of death. What they found confirmed the strong connection between foetal development and later risk of cardiovascular disease, and also gave strong clues as to why.

The men with the highest rates of death from cardiovascular disease were those who were thin at birth, where the placenta was low in weight, and where the mother was short and fat. Professor Barker explains this finding in the following way. If a mother is grossly undernourished during her own foetal development and infancy she will grow up to be shorter. As her nutrition improves in adulthood she gains weight, but not height, so she ends up short and fat. Her ability to produce a large, healthy placenta (the network of blood vessels that nourishes her offspring during pregnancy) is more dependent on her own early development, not just her level of nutrition during pregnancy. So her offspring will not have as good a supply of nutrients during its foetal development, despite her own improved nutrition. As a consequence, her baby is more likely to be short and thin, indicating poor foetal nutrition, and will have a greater risk of contracting diabetes and cardiovascular disease later in life. Conversely, a taller, well-nourished mother giving birth to a chubby baby means minimal risk of cardiovascular disease later in life.

SURVIVAL OF THE FATTEST

But what exactly is going on in the womb that programs disease decades later? The theory is that the developing foetus adapts to the inadequate nutrition by changing its metabolism and organ structure, favouring protection of the developing brain. This means that the infant is effectively born with insulin-resistance, as explained in Chapter 8. This altered metabolism of glucose and resistance to insulin programs the infant to develop blood sugar and cardiovascular problems later in life. While this theory is not yet proven, it is consistent with what is known about the offspring of pregnant animals who are malnourished.

Of course, if you happen to have been born small and thin, to a mother who was short and fat, this news may not be exactly welcome. However, we now know that a specific nutrition strategy, including the right balance of protein and carbohydrate, plus key amino acids, vitamins and minerals (see Chapter 8), may be able to reprogram the metabolism to reduce the risk of insulin-resistance. Also, knowing this, ensuring that infants born short and thin in relation to their gestational age receive the correct diet early on may have a significant effect in reducing the risk of cardiovascular disease later in life.

NUTRITIONAL ENVIRONMENT IS MORE IMPORTANT THAN GENES

What we are learning is that the environment to which we are exposed, especially the nutritional environment during foetal development, is more important that any inherited genes. Even those with a genetic predisposition, or an inherited predisposition due to a poor nutritional environment during foetal development, can decrease their risk through nutritional intervention. There is something positive that you can do to change the quality and length of your life.

....

CHAPTER 12

HOW TO GET HEART DISEASE – GUARANTEED RESULTS

After years of confusing, conflicting, complicated research and theories, we are starting to see the light at the end of the tunnel. A clear picture of how cardiovascular disease develops is emerging. With the knowledge of what you need to do to get heart disease, all that is necessary is to flip the card to know how to prevent and reverse the situation.

The story starts before birth, ends with premature death and goes like this:

1. Inherit the genes that predispose you to producing lipoprotein (a) and homocysteine.

2. Be born short and skinny to a short, overweight mother, thereby developing insulin-resistance.

3. Eat a refined food diet deficient in vitamin C, B6, B12 and folic acid, thereby increasing your levels of lipoprotein (a) and homocysteine.

4. Expose yourself to plenty of oxidants from fried and burnt food, smoking, pollution and exhaust fumes.

5. Eat a diet deficient in antioxidant nutrients, such as beta-carotene and vitamins C and E, by avoiding fruit and vegetables, nuts and seeds.

6. Eat plenty of saturated fat from meat, dairy produce and battery eggs and be deficient in essential fats from carnivorous fish, nuts and seeds.

7. Eat plenty of sugar, drink too much alcohol, avoid exercise and stay stressed.

8. Raise your blood pressure by eating salted and high-sodium foods, while avoiding fruits and vegetables which are rich in magnesium and potassium.

Do all this and you can reliably expect to have cardiovascular disease at a young age. On the other hand, if you eliminate as many of these factors as possible, you can expect to lead a long and healthy life, free from cardiovascular and related diseases, adding at least ten, if not 20, years to your healthy lifespan. Part 3 shows how to assess and reduce your risk.

HOW HEALTHY IS YOUR HEART?

CHAPTER 13

....

WHAT ARE THE RISK FACTORS?

There is no doubt that there are many contributive causes of cardiovascular disease, most of which can be eliminated by changing your diet and lifestyle. As the following stories illustrate, changing both is the secret, rather than relying on one factor to save your life (such as exercise or a low-cholesterol diet).

Jim Fix, the famous author of the *Complete Book of Running* died at the age of 52 from a heart attack while jogging. The autopsy found that two of his coronary arteries were almost totally clogged, which was not surprising to those who knew of his disregard for dietary advice. On the other hand, the heart surgeon, Dr Albert Starr, an advocator and follower of the low-cholesterol diet, needed open-heart surgery at only 47 years of age, the very same operation he had himself performed over 3000 times! In an experiment designed to determine which was more important – diet or exercise – Bill Solomon, from the University of Arizona, got some obliging pigs to run around a track, but fed them the average vitamin-deficient diet. Another group ate the pig-equivalent of healthfood but had no exercise; and a third group had both exercise *and* good nutrition. The third group of pigs fared best, proving that exercise and good nutrition together are vital for a healthy heart.

The many risk factors associated with heart disease are shown in the table below. You don't have to have all of them to be at risk. Smoking a little, drinking a little, exercising too little, eating a little too much fat and not enough protective vitamins and minerals can be as bad as smoking a lot or drinking a lot, provided other areas of your health are well covered. Later on in this chapter you'll be able to assess your overall risk and see clearly which changes to your diet and lifestyle will make the most difference to the health of your cardiovascular system. But, before assessing your risk, you need to understand why these factors are important.

Heart Disease Risk Factors

Lifestyle
Lack of aerobic exercise
Too much stress
Obesity
Smoking
Inherited predisposition

Test Results
High blood cholesterol (low HDL, high LDL)
High blood fats (triglycerides)
High blood pressure
High blood homocysteine
High lipoprotein (a)
Insulin-resistance

Diet
Too much dietary saturated fat
Too much sugar
Too many stimulants (tea, coffee)
Too much salt (sodium)
Too much alcohol
Too little antioxidant vitamins C and E
Too little B vitamins
Too little potassium, magnesium and calcium intake
Too little Omega 3 fats (fish and seeds)
Too little fresh fruit and vegetables

THE MAIN RISK FACTORS

Lack of Exercise

Human beings are designed to exercise. Just being sedentary doubles your risk of heart disease. Even moderate exercise two or three times a week has been shown to raise 'good' HDLs, lower cholesterol and blood pressure. One study by Wiley and associates found that even a hand-gripping exercise performed for two minutes, three times a week, for eight weeks, lowered blood pressure significantly. However, when the exercises were stopped for five weeks blood pressure returned to normal.[56]

The more you exercise, the stronger the effect. The most health-promoting exercises are 'aerobic', such as jogging, swimming, cycling and brisk walking. If you consider yourself unfit you'll need to start gently, perhaps exercising twice a week, for half an hour. Every 1.6km (1 mile) you walk or run theoretically gives you an extra 21 minutes of life and saves you 20 pence in medical care.[57] Therefore 1.6km (1 mile) a day for 20 years will add 106 days to your life and save you £1400. Get some good advice from a professional, so you don't start off with too ambitious an exercise schedule only to give up after a couple of weeks.

Stress

Stress promotes high blood pressure. This is a natural consequence of our evolutionary design. Our primate ancestors, when under stress, needed to 'fight or take flight'. One of the many changes that occur when we are under stress is the increase in our blood pressure necessary for the extreme muscular activity needed to fight or run. Another is the thickening of our blood, which would have helped heal wounds. Nowadays we rarely need to respond physically to the cause of stress, yet our blood pressure still increases and our blood still thickens. There is no doubt that prolonged stress increases the risk of heart disease, while acute stress can increase the risk of a heart attack.

According to recent research from the Department of Psychiatry and Behavioural Sciences at Duke University in

North Carolina, feelings of tension, frustration, sadness and hostility, which often result from the mental stresses of life, can more than double the risk of a heart attack in the hour immediately following a stressful event.[58] Although it isn't that easy to do, reducing stress and learning how to relax make a difference. Meditation, for example, has been proved to reduce high blood pressure, blood cholesterol and the risk of cardiovascular disease.[59] If you can't avoid stress then it's doubly important to make sure your nutrition is up to scratch.

Obesity

More than one-third of women and almost half of men are overweight. Being overweight is clearly associated with raised blood pressure, raised blood cholesterol and insulin-resistance or diabetes. Many of the causes of obesity (too much saturated fat and sugar, not enough nutrients, too little exercise) are also causes of cardiovascular disease. Reducing your weight so that it is the ideal range for your height by making positive changes to your diet and lifestyle will substantially reduce your risk.

Smoking

Smoking a packet of cigarettes a day gives you twice the risk of a heart attack and five times the risk of a stroke. Smoking 40 cigarettes a day means you are five times more likely to die of heart disease. In Britain 30,000 people die of heart disease each year as a direct result of smoking. The two major toxins in cigarettes are carbon monoxide and nicotine. Both increase blood clotting, promote artery damage and the formation of clots. Cigarettes also cause a restriction of blood vessels, therefore raising blood pressure. Nine out of ten heavy smokers have moderate to advanced atherosclerosis compared to three in ten non-smokers.

Inherited Risk

Some families have a very high incidence of cardiovascular disease at a young age. In some cases this may be due to inherited genes that, for example, predispose a person to producing lipoprotein (a) or homocysteine. In others, it may be the result of sub-optimum nutrition during pregnancy, passing on the tendency to insulin-resistance from generation to generation. However, in most cases, inherited risk is simply the inheritance of the same bad dietary and lifestyle habits. The good news is that you can rewrite history and change your risk by following the advice in this book, even if you've inherited the genetic predisposition to cardiovascular disease.

The Three Ss – Sugar, Saturated Fat and Stimulants

Sugar consumption is associated with both raised blood pressure and an increased incidence of cardiovascular disease. Some researchers even consider it to be more significant than the consumption of fat. Sugar increases blood stickiness which can lead to the formation of clots and increases resistance to insulin. Both excess insulin and raised blood sugar have damaging effects on the arteries.

If the extra sugar is not required it is converted into fat. A high sugar diet raises your blood pressure, decreases your resistance to stress (another risk factor in itself), and is associated with diabetes. Since most diabetics develop cardiovascular disease, the association between sugar, refined carbohydrates and heart disease is very strong. Conversely, a diet high in fibre and complex carbohydrates, such as lentils, beans and wholegrains, decreases your risk.

Sugar acts as a stimulant. It can induce bursts of hyperactivity followed by a slump in energy. So can other stimulants, like chocolate, cola drinks, coffee and tea, which stimulate the body to release sugar stores. Coffee and tea deplete the body of minerals, including potassium and magnesium, both by decreasing their absorption from food and by promoting their excretion via the kidneys. Cutting back on stimulants decreases your risk of cardiovascular disease.

Fat makes up 42 per cent of the calories in the average diet – and nearly half of that is saturated. Saturated fat is not an essential component of our diets, even though it is impossible and unnecessary to avoid it completely. It can be turned into glucose for energy or stored as fat which at least keeps us insulated and gives us padding. However it is healthier to cut down overall intake to 30 per cent of total calories, with saturated fat making up no more than one-third of that.

The old advice of switching from saturated fats to polyunsaturated fats, by, for example, eating margarine rather than butter, is not recommended. Polyunsaturated fats, when cooked or processed (as in margarine), lead to the formation of oxidants that damage cells in artery walls. So the message is to cut down on overall fat intake by having skimmed milk, becoming semi-vegetarian and eating fish and chicken instead of meat, having less cheese, and avoiding fast foods and heavily processed foods which are usually full of sugar and saturated fat. Foods rich in unprocessed polyunsaturated fats are beneficial to the body and are best eaten raw. So keep your cold-pressed vegetable oils for salad dressings and mayonnaise, eat nuts and seeds, and avoid frying as much as you can.

Salt

Salt is a preservative. It first came into use to preserve meat by slowing down the enzyme reactions that cause meat to decay. Although you need to take in some salt every day it is present in all foods, including fruit and vegetables. There is simply no need to add it to your diet. The excessive consumption of salt is known to raise blood pressure, especially in susceptible individuals. Unfortunately, there is no easy way to determine whether or not you are particularly susceptible to the effects of salt so the best advice is to avoid added salt. The average person consumes over 10g a day which is more than 20 times our actual requirement. For most people, avoiding salt makes a measurable difference to blood pressure.

Alcohol

Small amounts of alcohol may actually be good for you. Studies have shown that a small daily intake of alcohol actually raises levels of HDLs, which help to return cholesterol to the liver from where it can be excreted from the body. Red wine, rich in antioxidant proanthocyanidins, is particularly beneficial. So a maximum of one glass of wine *may* be beneficial. However, even small amounts of alcohol seem to raise blood pressure.

A group of researchers wondered why people going into hospital tended to experience a drop in blood pressure. Thinking that the reduction in alcohol consumption might have something to do with it, they equipped a new group of patients with a complementary daily can of beer. Sure enough, these patients didn't show the usual decline in blood pressure. Alcohol, being a neurotoxin, and a substance which robs the body of both vitamins and minerals, can hardly be recommended for improving your health. However, a glass of red wine a day, at least from the point of view of heart disease, probably has little negative effect and may be beneficial.

THE MAIN PROTECTORS

Vitamins and Minerals

The role of vitamins and minerals in preventing cardiovascular disease is greatly underestimated. It is hard to know to what extent the decline in our intake of vitamins and minerals has been responsible for the increase in cardiovascular disease. A good supply of antioxidant nutrients, which protect the body from harmful free radicals that damage cells in the artery wall, is essential.

Vitamin A (both retinol, the animal form, and beta-carotene, the vegetable form), vitamin C and E all act as antioxidants. Other antioxidant enzymes depend upon selenium and zinc. Vitamin B6, folic acid and B12 deficiency are also associated with cardiovascular disease, largely because they prevent the formation of homocysteine which damages arteries. Blood pressure can be lowered by ensuring a good intake of calcium, magnesium and potassium. Of these, magnesium is the most important nutrient. The role all these nutrients play in preventing cardiovascular disease is explained fully, together with recommended intakes, in Part 4.

Fish Oils

Fish Oils are rich in Omega 3 fats and also provide protection against cardiovascular disease. Foods rich in these fats are seeds such as pumpkin and flax, or carnivorous fish such as salmon, herring, mackerel and tuna. An alternative is to take fish oil supplements, a concentrated source of the Omega 3 fats EPA and DHA. Like all essential fats, frying these fish damages the oils, making them less beneficial.

Fruit and Vegetables

If you're not eating your greens, reds, yellows and blues your cardiovascular risk is higher. The natural colours in fruits and vegetables are antioxidants, protecting against arterial damage. Fruits and vegetables are also rich in the vitamins and minerals that protect against heart disease, especially potassium and magnesium. The more we learn about the hundreds of beneficial 'phytonutrients' in plants, the more we understand why eating five servings of fruits and vegetables a day is associated with a high degree of protection from heart disease.

THE BEST PREDICTORS

Your Cholesterol and Fat Profile

The best predictor of heart disease is the level of cholesterol and triglycerides in your blood. In order to be carried in the blood, cholesterol becomes bound to a type of protein called a lipoprotein. Usually, around 70 per cent of the cholesterol in the blood is carried in the form of low-density lipoproteins (LDLs). The rest is carried in the form of high-density lipoproteins (HDLs).

As overall blood cholesterol levels rise, so does the amount of LDLs, both of which indicate an increased risk for cardiovascular disease. HDLs, on the other hand, seem to help remove cholesterol from the blood and from artery walls. So a raised HDL level is, broadly speaking, consistent with a reduced risk. The best predictor is the ratio between total cholesterol and HDL cholesterol (see the table on page 22).

Lipoprotein (a) is a specific lipoprotein that encourages arterial blockage (see Chapter 7). A high level is a reliable predictor of risk, so it's good to know your level. Also worth knowing is your homocysteine level (see Chapter 9). Again, high levels indicate an increased risk. A high level of triglycerides in the blood (see the table on page 29) also indicates an increased risk.

Your Pulse and Blood Pressure

Your pulse and blood pressure are the easiest way to get some insight into the health of your cardiovascular system. Your pulse reflects the strength of your heart. If your heart only has to beat 60 times each minute to get the blood circulating around your body it is obviously healthier than if your heart has to beat 80 times a minute. The more you exercise, the stronger your heart (which is, after all, just a muscle) becomes. Cyclists have very large hearts, while sedentary people have small hearts. The ideal pulse rate is below 65 beats a minute. Some athletes have pulse rates as low as 45; however, for most of us, getting down to 60 is the most we can hope for.

Your blood pressure reflects the health of your arteries more than the health of your heart. The higher your blood pressure, the more likely you are to have atherosclerosis and the greater your risk of cardiovascular disease. Generally speaking, a systolic pressure above 140, or a diastolic pressure above 90 indicates a significant risk for heart disease. The table on page 11 shows you the blood pressure and pulse readings for low, medium and high risk.

CHAPTER 14

....

THE HEALTHY HEART
CHECK

The following questionnaires will help you assess your rating for each of the major risk factors. The central diagram represents the diameter of an artery. For each point you score, shade in one of the blocks, starting from the outer edge – this will give you an at-a-glance view of your risk of heart disease. The greater your risk, the smaller the diameter of the artery, leaving less room for the blood to flow with a higher chance of blockages. The more blocked a section is, the more important it is to make some changes in this area of your diet and lifestyle.

In both questionnaires, if you shade beyond the embold-ened inner circle in any section it means that this area warrants your attention. If you end up with less than ten unshaded sections I recommend you seek the guidance of a nutrition consultant who can help you devise an effective strategy to improve your health and reduce your risk of disease.

Diet and Lifestyle Questionnaire

If you answer 'yes' to any of these questions, shade one section, starting from the outer edge, in the chart:

1. Vitamins and Minerals
    a. Do you rarely take vitamin supplements?
    b. Do you rarely take extra vitamin C or E?

    c. Do you often eat less than two servings of fruit and vegetables a day?

    d. Do you add salt to your cooking and food?

2. Stress and Stimulants

    a. Do you consider your lifestyle very stressful?

    b. Do you feel guilty when relaxing and get angry easily?

    c. Do you eat more than 1 tablespoonful of sugar each day, in drinks, chocolate or sugary snacks?

    d. Do you drink coffee or tea at regular intervals during the day?

3. Smoking and Drinking

    a. Do you smoke more than five cigarettes a day?

    b. Do you smoke more than 20 cigarettes a day?

    c. Do you have alcohol every day?

    d. Do you have more than two alcoholic drinks a day?

4. Health – Past and Present

    a. Have you ever had a stroke, heart attack or thrombosis?

    b. Were you small at birth and was your mother short and overweight?

    c. Have either of your parents ever had cardiovascular disease or diabetes?

    d. Do you have any history of high blood pressure?

5. Exercise and Obesity

    a. Do you exercise for less than 20 minutes twice a week?

    b. Do you consider yourself unfit?

    c. Are you more than 7kg (14lb) over your ideal weight?

    d. Are you more than 10kg (22lb) over your ideal weight?

6. Dietary Fat

    a. Do you eat red meat more than three times per week?

    b. Do you eat fried foods more than twice per week?

    c. Do you rarely eat oily fish (tuna, mackeral etc.)?

    d. Do you rarely eat nuts and seeds?

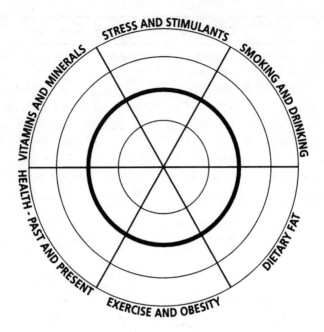

Fig 11 – If you answer 'yes' to any of the questions on pages 82–3, shade one section, starting from the outer edge of the chart

Cardiovascular Statistics Questionnaire

If the following statistics apply to you, shade one section, starting from the outer edge, in the Cardiovascular chart. The more blocked a section, the more important it is to make some changes in your diet and lifestyle.

	Outer ring	Middle ring	Inner ring
Blood pressure	>120/80	>135/85	>140/90
Cholesterol	>5.18mmol/l or >200mg%	>6.2mmol/l or >240mg%	>6.7mmol/l or >260mg%
Triglycerides	>1mmol/l or >89mg%	>1.5mmol/l or >133mg%	>1.95mmol/l or >173mg%
Cholesterol/HDL ratio	>3:1	>5:1	>8:1
Lipoprotein(a)	>10mg/dl	>20mg/dl	>30mg/dl
Homocysteine	>10µmol/l	>13µmol/l	>16µmol/l

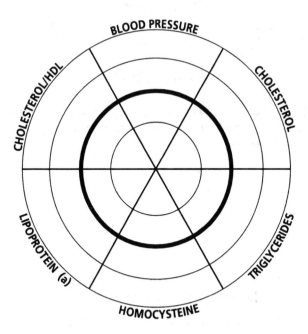

Fig 12 – If the above statistics apply to you, shade one section, starting from the outer edge, in the Cardiovascular chart

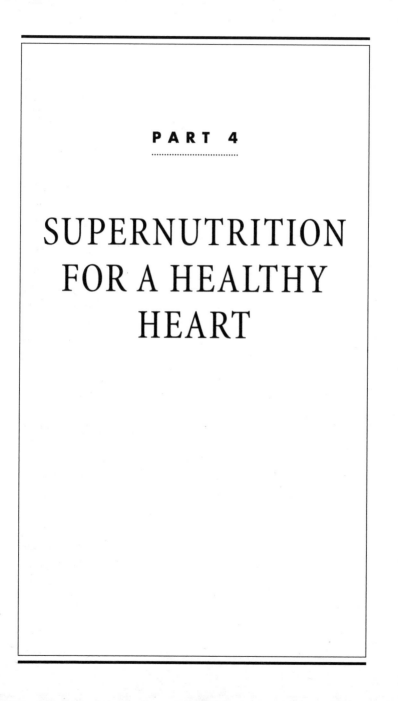

PART 4

SUPERNUTRITION FOR A HEALTHY HEART

....

CHAPTER 15

THE ACE PROTECTORS

A major breakthrough in heart disease went unnoticed on 21 March 1996. The results of the first large-scale, double-blind, controlled trial on vitamin E supplements, carried out by Professor Morris Brown and colleagues at Cambridge University were published. They proved a 75 per cent decrease in death or heart attack in a group of 2000 patients with heart disease, compared to those on a placebo.[60] These results are approximately three times better than any drug yet tested. Professor Morris Brown said, 'This is even more exciting than aspirin. Most people in our study were already taking aspirin. The average benefit from taking aspirin is in the order of 25 to 30 per cent reduction. Vitamin E reduces the risk of heart attack by a massive 75 per cent.'

This was the third large-scale trial to prove the cardiovascular benefits of taking vitamin E supplements. In one study, published in 1993 in the *New England Journal of Medicine*, 87, 200 nurses were given 100iu of vitamin E daily for more than two years.[61] A 40 per cent drop in fatal and non-fatal heart attacks was reported amongst the subjects, compared to those not taking vitamin E. In the other study 39,000 male health professionals were given 100iu of vitamin E for the same length of time; they experienced a 39 per cent reduction in heart attacks.[62]

Reading these results, you might wonder why on earth

doctors aren't prescribing vitamin E for every patient with a risk of cardiovascular disease, and why we aren't all taking vitamin E supplements. Good question.

THE VITAMIN E STORY

In truth, the value of vitamin E was already known by Dr Evan Shute half a century ago, in 1948. This eminent physician dedicated his life to researching and publicising the value of vitamin E in preventing heart disease and saving lives. Far from giving him any accolades for this important discovery, cardiologists tried to shut him down. A group of US cardiologists went before the Postmaster General and pleaded for vitamin E to be banned from the US mail. One cardiologist after another testified that vitamin E was worthless in treating any form of human disease. One compared it to snake oil. The result was that vitamin E was *banned* from the US mail. The only place you could buy it was the Shute Foundation in Canada, and if you wanted to take it out of the country it had to be smuggled to avoid confiscation by customs officials.

Fifty years on, despite the fact that the evidence for vitamin E is rock solid, the medical profession is still dragging its heels. Even Professor Brown, who now recommends that those with heart disease take 400 to 800iu of vitamin E a day, said, 'It would be irresponsible for us to recommend it freely to those without heart disease.' In other words, wait until you're at risk. This, he says, is because his group's research proved that vitamin E protects those *with* heart disease, but didn't assess its protective value for those without. Fair enough. Yet the consistent results of other trials giving vitamin E to those not at risk confirm that it gives significant protection.

For example, a ten-year study, involving 11,178 people aged 67 to 105, found that those supplementing vitamin E had a reduced risk of death from all causes of 33 per cent, and a reduced risk of 47 per cent of dying from heart attacks. Those who used vitamin E for longer periods of time reduced their risk of death from cancer and heart disease to less than half that of those who didn't take supplements. Taking both vitamin C and vitamin E supplements reduced overall risk of death by 42 per cent and the risk of death from a heart attack by 52 per cent.[63] We could save billions of pounds per year in healthcare costs by acting on this information.

How Much is Enough?

However, not all research trials have confirmed vitamin E's preventive powers. In a recent trial, reported in the *Lancet*, smokers aged 50 to 69, who had had a heart attack, were given a daily supplement of 50mg of vitamin E and 20mg beta-carotene. This level of supplementation gave no extra protection from their second heart attack.

According to Dr Diaz and colleagues at the Evans Memorial Department of Medicine and the Whitaker Cardiovascular Institute at the Boston University School of Medicine, this study is more the exception than the rule and indicates the importance of dosage. They comprehensively reviewed all the human studies on vitamin E and concluded that there is ample evidence that vitamin E does reduce cardiovascular risk.[64]

As both Dr Evan Shute and Professor Morris Brown found, you have to take sufficiently high levels of vitamin E and you have to take it for an extended period of time to get positive results. Studies show that giving less than 100mg doesn't always have any effect. The protection given seems to increase as the daily intake rises from 100 to 400mg, though taking in levels above 400mg offers diminishing returns.

Professor Morris Brown found no difference in benefit between those taking 400 and 800mg. Dr Evan Shute recommended between 300 and 700mg (equivalent to between 400 and 1000iu) per day. He also found that no significant protection was achieved until a person had taken the vitamin supplement for six months. The longer they took it, the more protection it conferred. Again, Professor Brown's research found the same thing. The difference in the number of heart attacks, between those taking vitamin E and those on a placebo, only became apparent after the first 200 days of the trial.

Another benefit of supplementing vitamin E is in treating intermittent claudication (pain and lameness in the limbs caused by arterial blockage). In a double-blind study, 1600mg daily of vitamin E reduced this important and painful symptom of cardiovascular disease by 66 per cent.[65]

How Do Antioxidants Work?

Antioxidants work by disarming harmful oxidants (free radicals) – molecules that can damage cholesterol and fat travelling through the arteries, as well as the artery wall itself. Vitamin E (technically known as d-alpha tocopherol) is a fat-soluble antioxidant and, as such, can help to protect fats such as cholesterol. If cholesterol and fat are damaged as they travel through arteries, they can build up within arterial cells, overloading them until they are known as foam cells. These can change their pattern of behaviour, multiplying somewhat like a cancer cell and forming a growing wound on the wall of the artery which encourages inflammation and blood clots.

To help deal with inflammation, the body produces nitric oxide. Yet, in the presence of oxidants, like cigarette smoke or fried food, the nitric oxide is converted into peroxinitrate, which can further damage the artery wall. A relative of vitamin E, gamma tocopherol (which is also found in vitamin E rich foods such as seeds, nuts and wheatgerm), is actually better at protecting nitric oxide than vitamin E itself. According to Dr Stephan Christen, a medical researcher from Cleveland,

Ohio, who specialises in vitamin E, 'People who take higher doses of vitamin E supplements with only alpha-tocopherol may not be realising the full benefit, as compared with supplements which also contain gamma-tocopherol.' For this reason some supplement companies provide natural vitamin E (d–alpha tocopherol) together with other tocopherols, including gamma tocopherol.

The ideal daily intake is probably between 200mg (300iu) and 400mg (600iu). However, taking supplements isn't the same as eating a diet naturally rich in vitamin E, other tocopherols and many important phytonutrients. The best foods for vitamin E are shown in the table below. Given that a daily dietary intake of more than 50mg is very hard to achieve, there is clearly value in taking vitamin E supplements on top of a vitamin E rich diet.

Which Foods are Best for Vitamin E?

Foods are listed in order of those that contain the most vitamin E per calorie of food. The figures in brackets are the amount of vitamin E in 100g, which is roughly equivalent to a cup or serving.

Cold-pressed seed oil	(83mg)	Salmon	(1.8mg)
Sunflower seeds	(52.6mg)	Sweet potato	(4.0mg)
Peanuts	(11.8mg)	Almonds	(24.5mg)
Sesame seeds	(22.7mg)	Walnuts	(19.6mg)
Beans	(7.7mg)	Pecans	(19.8mg)
Peas	(2.3mg)	Cashews	(10.9mg)
Wheatgerm	(27.5mg)	Brown rice	(2.0mg)
Tuna	(6.3mg)	Lentils	(1.3mg)
Sardines	(2.0mg)		

THE ROLE OF VITAMIN C

The next most important antioxidant vitamin is vitamin C. Being water-soluble, it helps to clean up oxidants in 'watery' parts of the body; so, working with vitamin E, all territories are covered. In fact, vitamin C can recycle vitamin E. If a molecule of vitamin C disarms an oxidant and becomes inactivated, it is reactivated if it meets a vitamin E molecule. The same is true for vitamin E, which is probably why the combination of vitamin C and E has proved so effective in trials, halving the risk of a heart attack.

Vitamin C Lowers Blood Pressure

Vitamin C also lowers high blood pressure. A number of studies have shown that the higher a person's vitamin C status, the lower their blood pressure.[66] In one double-blind study, participants were given 1000mg (1g) of vitamin C or a placebo and researchers found significant reduction in the systolic blood pressure, but not the diastolic. The research group, from the Alcorn State University in Mississippi, concluded that, 'Vitamin C supplementation may have therapeutic value in human hypertensive disease.'[67] The ability of vitamin C, at a daily level of 1g, to lower blood pressure, as well as cholesterol levels, has been demonstrated in other studies as well.[68]

Vitamin C's main role in reducing cardiovascular risk may be its ability to lower lipoprotein (a) (discussed in Chapter 7), high levels of which are a major risk factor for heart disease. Vitamin C deficiency leads to arterial damage, eventually resulting in bleeding, which is the sign of scurvy. It is important not only to have enough vitamin C to prevent these defects but also to have extra, if there is already arterial damage, in order to remove unwanted lipoprotein deposits and help rebuild the artery wall.

Which Foods are Best for Vitamin C?

Foods are listed in order of those that contain the most vitamin C per calorie of food. The figures in brackets are the amount of vitamin C in 100g, which is roughly equivalent to a cup or serving.

Peppers	(100mg)	Papayas	(62mg)
Watercress	(60mg)	Peas	(25mg)
Cabbage	(60mg)	Melons	(25mg)
Broccoli	(110mg)	Oranges	(50mg)
Cauliflower	(60mg)	Grapefruits	(40mg)
Strawberries	(60mg)	Limes	(29mg)
Lemons	(80mg)	Tomatoes	(60mg)
Kiwi fruit	(85mg)	Tangerines	(31mg)
Brussels sprouts	(62mg)	Mangoes	(28mg)

For prevention of cardiovascular disease, an ideal intake of vitamin C starts at 1g a day. That's the equivalent of 22 oranges. A survey of doctors found that the healthiest consumed a diet that provided 410mg of vitamin C, which is about the maximum you're going to get if you eat five servings of fruits and vegetables a day. On top of this, it may well be worth supplementing 1g as a minimum and 5g if you have a high risk of cardiovascular disease.

HOW IMPORTANT IS VITAMIN A?

The evidence for supplementing the antioxidant vitamin A, or rather its precursor beta-carotene, is less convincing. In the Nurses' Health Study in which 121,000 US female nurses aged 30 to 55 were monitored, those who consumed more than 15–20mg of beta-carotene a day had a 40 per cent lower risk of stroke and 22 per cent lower risk of heart attack, compared to women who reported eating less than 6mg a day.[69] In Switzerland a 12-year follow-up study of those who had died from cardiovascular disease found that there was double the risk of death from a heart attack or stroke in those who initially had low blood levels of beta-carotene (below 12 mcg%).[70]

While these studies do suggest that a good dietary intake and high blood levels of beta-carotene equate to a lower risk of cardiovascular disease, the results of supplementation haven't been as encouraging as those of vitamin E and C. Beta-carotene is, however, very protective against cancer. I therefore recommend eating a diet that provides 18mg (10,000iu) of beta-carotene as well as supplementing 18mg a day.

Which Foods are Best for Beta-Carotene?

Foods are listed in order of those that contain the most beta-carotene per calorie of food. The figures in brackets are the amount of beta-carotene in 100g, which is roughly equivalent to a cup or serving.

Beef liver	(35,778iu)	Broccoli	(1541iu)
Veal liver	(26,562iu)	Apricots (fresh)	(2612iu)
Carrots	(28,125iu)	Papayas	(2014iu)
Watercress	(4700iu)	Asparagus	(829iu)
Cabbage	(3000iu)	Apricots (dried)	(7240iu)
Squash	(7000iu)	Peppers	(530iu)
Sweet potatoes	(17,055iu)	Tangerines	(920iu)
Melon	(3224iu)	Nectarines	(730iu)
Pumpkin	(1600iu)	Peaches	(535iu)
Mangoes	(3894iu)	Watermelon	(365iu)
Tomatoes	(1133iu)		

ALL-ROUND ANTIOXIDANT PROTECTION

There is little doubt that the best way to get all-round antioxidant protection is to eat a diet rich in natural antioxidants and take an all-round antioxidant supplement. The best all-round foods to eat are shown below. These not only contain vitamins A, C and E, but also contain many other key antioxidant

Antioxidants – the Best Foods

The best all-round antioxidant foods have the highest numbers of stars. Foods are listed in order of their star rating. Make sure these foods form a large part of your diet.

Food	Rich Source of		
	A	C	E
Sweet potatoes	★★★	★	★★★
Carrots	★★★	★★★	
Watercress	★★★	★★★	
Peas	★	★★	★★
Broccoli	★★	★★★	
Cauliflower	★	★★★	
Lemons	★	★★★	
Mangoes	★★	★★	
Meat	★★		★★
Melon	★★	★★	
Peppers	★	★★★	
Pumpkin	★★	★★	
Strawberries	★	★★★	
Tomatoes	★★	★★	
Cabbage	★★★		
Grapefruit	★	★★	
Kiwi fruit	★	★★	
Oranges	★	★★	
Seeds and nuts			★★★
Squash	★★★		
Tuna, mackerel, salmon			★★★
Wheatgerm			★★★
Apricots	★★		
Beans			★★

Fig 13 – The ACE foods to Include in Your Diet

nutrients such as proanthocyanidins, lycopene, glutathione, cysteine and more. So the golden rule is to eat at least five servings of fresh fruit and vegetables a day and make sure your diet is naturally multi-coloured. Green, red, yellow and blue foods all provide a varied and rich supply of antioxidants to fight off the oxidant artery invaders.

The Ideal Antioxidant Supplement

	Antioxidant	Multivitamin plus C	Suggested daily amount
Vitamin A, as retinol	5000iu (1.5mgRE)	5000iu (3mgRE)	10,000iu (3mgRE)
Vitamin A, as beta-carotene	5000iu (1.5mgRE)	5000iu (1.5mgRE)	10,000iu (3mgRE)*
Vitamin C	500mg	1500mg	2000mg
Vitamin E	200mg	200mg	400mg
Reduced glutathione	50mg		50mg
or N-acetyl cysteine	500mg		500mg
Proanthocyanidins (e.g. bilberry, grape seed)	100mg		100mg
Pycnogenol (from pine)	5mg		5mg
Silymarin (from milk thistle)	100mg		100mg
Selenium	100mcg	50mcg	150mcg
Zinc	5mg	10mg	15mg
Manganese	2mg	3mg	5mg
Iron		10mg	10mg
Copper		0.5mg	0.5mg

* This is equivalent to supplementing 18mg of beta-carotene

As far as antioxidant supplements are concerned, those listed in the chart on page 97 are the ingredients to look for. It isn't necessary to have every one of these antioxidant substances, but a decent antioxidant will contain all the antioxidant vitamins and amino acids, plus some plant-based antioxidants. The levels given are approximate guides only and may equate to taking two or three antioxidant complexes a day. Levels much lower than these are likely to be ineffective.

The suggested daily amounts are the sum of what you can obtain from an antioxidant supplement, plus a high-strength multivitamin and multimineral, plus 1000mg of vitamin C (discussed fully in Chapter 7).

Since vitamin C is rarely supplied in sufficient amounts, you will need to take a good high-strength antioxidant formula and additional vitamin C. It may also be preferable not to supplement the minerals iron, copper, zinc and manganese, together with glutathione, since they compete. Vitamin E and vitamin C protect each other. So do reduced glutathione and anthocyanidins (also called anthocyans), making them a good combination.

CHAPTER 16

EPA – THE ESKIMO SECRET

While too much saturated fat (predominantly found in meat and dairy produce) is clearly bad news as far as heart disease and general health is concerned, essential fats are good news. We learnt, in Chapter 6, of the benefits of both the Omega 3 and Omega 6 family of fats, but especially of the Omega 3 fish oils.

It was this discovery of the numerous benefits of Omega 3 fish oils that led to the understanding that the Inuit and the Japanese were achieving significant protection from cardio-vascular disease by eating large quantities of fish.

Fish isn't the only source of Omega 3 fats, although it is the most effective. These Omega 3 fats originally come from the vegetable kingdom – in the case of fish, from plankton that they eat. For us humans, the best dietary sources are seeds, especially flax (linseed) and certain strains of pumpkin. Generally speaking, the colder the climate, the richer the seeds are in alpha linolenic acid (the main Omega 3 fat found in seeds). The linolenic acid is then converted in the body into EPA and DHA, types of Omega 3 fats that are especially rich in certain fish and have been found to be the most pro-tective against cardiovascular disease.

SEEDS AND THEIR OILS – HOW MUCH DO YOU NEED?

Since not all linolenic acid is converted into EPA and DHA (a process that depends on sufficient intake of vitamins B3 and C) you have to eat a lot of seeds to gain any measurable protection from cardiovascular disease. The ideal daily intake is a heaped tablespoon of seeds a day, or 15 ml (1 tablespoon) of seed oil. Since seeds are also very rich sources of calcium and magnesium (see Chapter 17), they are preferable to the oil, while both oil and seeds are a rich source of vitamin E.

To get the most benefit from seeds, it is best to grind them in a coffee grinder. Grind a mixture of equal amounts of flax, pumpkin, sunflower and sesame seeds (together providing the right balance of Omega 3 and Omega 6) and sprinkle a heaped tablespoon on your cereal in the morning; add seeds to soups, salads and other dishes. Seeds are best kept whole (unground) in a sealed jar in the fridge. This minimises exposure to heat, light and oxygen, keeping them fresher for longer.

There are also a number of excellent oil blends now available in healthfood stores. Look for ones that have equal quantities of Omega 3 and Omega 6 or a ratio of two parts Omega 3 to one part Omega 6. The best ones use cold-pressed, organic oils (e.g. a combination of flax, pumpkin, sesame, sunflower, borage, etc) in a light-proof bottle. As heat destroys these oils, you should never fry with them. Use them for salad dressings; on baked potatoes and cooked vegetables (instead of butter); add to a casserole or soup before serving; or even add to your cereal in the morning or take a spoonful as it is. The ideal intake, if you are not also eating seeds, is 15ml (1 tablespoon) a day.

OMEGA 3 FISH OILS – HOW MUCH DO YOU NEED?

Our modern diet and lifestyle are so far removed from those which we appear to be designed for, that it is increasingly difficult to get all the nutrients we need from a well-balanced diet alone.

Much of the food we eat has the nutrients processed out to increase its shelf-life and profitability. Even fresh foods often have lower nutrient content than they used to, due to over-farming and soil depletion. Pollution has introduced so-called 'anti-nutrients' into the air, the soil and the seas.

For this reason, many nutritionists recommend supplementing concentrated essential fatty acids, and particularly EPA. The amount you need depends on what you need it for. For simply preventing ill-health and maintaining healthy arteries, supple joints, good skin and mental function, 360mg of EPA is probably sufficient.

Smoking, drinking alcohol frequently, eating fried food and sources of saturated fat all 'block' the body's ability to process EPA and so may push up your requirement.

If you're interested in adding EPA to your diet because you have a risk of cardiovascular disease, have had a stroke or heart attack, or are suffering from high blood pressure or angina, then most trials have proved the benefit of daily doses of 1200 to 3000mg.

Capsules of EPA usually provide anywhere from 180mg to 400mg, so, if you choose the high-strength capsules, this means three to eight capsules a day. This equates to eating 100g of fish three to six times a week.

WHICH FISH SHOULD YOU EAT?

An alternative to taking capsules is to eat fish. The only drawback is pollution. The health of a fish depends largely on where it is caught – on the whole, the further away from coastal waters the better. Places like the English Channel are highly polluted, while the Arctic Ocean is not. The chart below gives the amount of Omega 3 fatty acids you'd expect to find in some commonly available fish. About 20 per cent of the Omega 3 fatty acids in these fish will be EPA, so you need to get about 6g of Omega 3s a week to reach the therapeutic level – that's the equivalent of eating 250g of mackerel a week. (Smoked salmon and smoked mackerel will give you the same benefits as fresh.)

Average Omega 3 Content in Fish

Fish (100g/3.5oz, uncooked)	Omega 3s (g)
Mackerel, Atlantic	2.5
Herring, Atlantic	1.7
Tuna, Bluefin	1.2
Salmon, Coho	1.0
Turbot (flatfish)	0.9
Bass, striped	0.8
Trout, rainbow	0.7
Shrimp	0.5
Halibut, Pacific	0.4
Flounder*/Sole	0.2

*Analysis on cooked fish

CHAPTER 17

DECREASE THE PRESSURE WITH MINERALS

One of the most effective ways to lower blood pressure is to change the balance of minerals in your diet. This is because the inner wall of the arteries contains a layer of muscle which is either relaxed or contracted, depending on the electrical difference of 'electrolytic' minerals inside and outside the muscle cells. When the muscle contracts, blood pressure increases. Contraction is a normal response to stress, as it helps get glucose from the blood into the cells. However, if this response goes on too long, or if the blood vessel concerned is already partially blocked, the result can be high blood pressure or even total blockage, triggering a heart attack or stroke.

THE ROLE OF MINERALS

The minerals calcium, magnesium and potassium all relax the arterial muscle, and sodium contracts it. If each of these first three are given in isolation, they significantly lower blood pressure, while avoiding sodium (found in salt, which is sodium chloride) has the same effect.[71] Of these, magnesium has the greatest effect (discussed in Chapter 10). While the effect of each mineral individually is less than that of the drugs commonly used to reduce blood pressure, a combined increase in calcium, magnesium and potassium intake, coupled with a decrease in sodium, can dramatically lower blood pressure within days – equivalent to or better than the drugs, but without the side-effects.[72]

Increasing calcium, magnesium and potassium has a much more profound effect on blood pressure than restricting sodium, alcohol or even dietary fat. The scale of protection is more akin to that given by taking regular exercise. Of course, any change would be greatest in those whose diets were deficient in calcium, magnesium and potassium and excessive in sodium.

The ideal intake of calcium is in the order of 800 to 1000mg a day. A study at the Oregon Health Sciences Institute by Dr McCarron and colleagues found that these levels of calcium lowered blood pressure. And a survey by Queen Elizabeth College, University of London, found that 73 per cent of women failed to achieve a dietary intake of 500mg.[73] In doses of up to 1200mg a day, there is a clear relationship between increasing calcium intake and decreasing blood pressure.[74] However, more is not necessarily better. Above 2000mg a day will impair your health (by stressing the kidneys), rather than improve it.[75]

Calcium, taken in a 1:1 ratio with magnesium, is most effective, balanced with a high intake of potassium.[76] Potassium is not worth supplementing since the highest dose available is 100mg. On the other hand, fresh fruit and vegetables or their juices can supply several thousand milligrams of potassium. Sodium restriction alone is most effective for those who are particularly salt-sensitive – around 10 per cent of the population.

Sodium is easily avoided by not adding salt to your food or eating foods containing salt. Calcium and magnesium are richest in seeds (sesame and sunflower) and nuts (almonds), while potassium is very rich in fruit and vegetables, which (especially root vegetables) are also good sources of magnesium and reasonable sources of calcium. Dairy products, although high in calcium, are a poor source of magnesium and are associated with an increase in cardiovascular disease, especially strokes.

Putting all this together into a diet high in fruit, vegetables, nuts and seeds, and low in salt, dairy produce and fat, lowers blood pressure as efficiently as hypertensive drug therapy, according to the Well Centre for Prevention and Clinical Research at Johns Hopkins University in the USA. Researchers there found that this kind of diet lowered systolic blood pressure (the top figure) by 11.4 points and diastolic by 5.5 points.[77] In all these minerals, magnesium is the most commonly deficient and it's well worth supplementing 400mg of both calcium and magnesium if you've got high blood pressure.

Which Foods are Best for Calcium, Magnesium and Potassium?

Foods are listed in order of those that contain the most mineral per calorie of food. The figures in brackets are the amount of the mineral in 100g, which is roughly equivalent to a cup or serving.

Calcium		Magnesium		Potassium	
Swiss cheese	(925mg)	Wheatgerm	(490mg)	Watercress	(329mg)
Cheddar cheese	(750mg)	Pumpkin seeds	(534mg)	Endive	(316mg)
Almonds	(234mg)	Almonds	(270mg)	Cabbage	(251mg)
Parsley	(203mg)	Cashews	(267mg)	Celery	(285mg)
Sesame seeds	(975mg)	Sunflower seeds	(354mg)	Courgette	(248mg)
Sunflower seeds	(116mg)	Sesame Seeds	(350mg)	Parsley	(540mg)
Pumpkin seeds	(51mg)	Buckwheat flour	(229mg)	Radishes	(231mg)
Cooked dried beans	(50mg)	Brazil nuts	(225mg)	Cauliflower	(355mg)
Wholewheat	(46mg)	Peanuts	(175mg)	Mushrooms	(371mg)
Broccoli	(68mg)	Pecan nuts	(142mg)	Pumpkin	(339mg)
Kale	(249mg)	Cooked beans	(37mg)	Molasses	(2925mg)
Tofu	(145mg)	Garlic	(36mg)	Broccoli	(325mg)
Milk	(120mg)	Raisins	(35mg)	Tomato	(207mg)
		Peas	(35mg)		

MULTINUTRIENT APPROACHES ARE EVEN BETTER

The best results of all, however, have been achieved by a more general strategy of a good diet, plus additional vitamin, mineral and essential fat supplements. Dr Michael Colgan, from the Colgan Institute of Nutritional Science, found just that. He put 33 people on a comprehensive vitamin and mineral programme and they all experienced a gradual decrease in both blood pressure and pulse rates over the next four years, irrespective of their age. The participants' average blood pressure dropped from slightly above 140/90 to below 120/80, while their pulse rates decreased from 76 to an average of 65 beats per minute over five years on nutritional supplements, such as those shown in the chart on page 13.

A short three-month trial involving 34 people with high blood pressure at the Institute for Optimum Nutrition in London achieved an average eight-point drop in systolic and diastolic blood pressure by supplementing vitamins, minerals and some EPA. The greatest decreases were in those with the highest initial blood pressure.

IRON – IS TOO MUCH DANGEROUS?

Iron is an important trace element needed primarily to carry oxygen in the body. It is also commonly deficient, with 1 per cent of men and 5 per cent of women suffering from anaemia, and an average intake of 10mg (compared to the RDA of 14mg). Yet startling new evidence suggests that too much iron may be as much of a cause for concern as too little, predisposing individuals to heart disease.

In one Finnish study of 1900 men, those with higher iron stores were more than twice as likely to have heart attacks.[78] In fact, excess iron was a greater risk factor than excess cholesterol. Jerome Sullivan, a pathologist at the Veterans

Affairs Medical Centre in Charleston, South Carolina, wondered why men had a higher risk than women, until after the menopause.[78] Another anomaly he noticed was that women who had undergone hysterectomies also had a higher heart disease rate. He found that ingested iron is converted into ferritin and is then very hard to eliminate. Men consuming excess iron accumulate it and, by the age of 45, have four times the iron levels of women. Women, on the other hand, lose iron through menstruation, until the menopause. By the age of 70, women have equal ferritin levels, and equal risks for heart disease. Further supportive evidence comes from analyses of men who donate blood. Giving blood lowers ferritin levels and decreases measures of risk for heart disease. A ferritin level above 150µg/l is considered suspect.

While the jury is still out on the true dangers of too much iron, we urge caution on excessive supplementation, especially among meat-eaters. Taking supplements of more than 15mg a day is not advisable, unless you have a known deficiency. Iron is also an antagonist of zinc (Britain's most deficient trace element) and both iron and zinc are involved in antioxidant protection for cholesterol. An excess of iron and deficiency of zinc may lead to 'oxidising' of cholesterol, thereby increasing heart disease risk.

CHAPTER 18

BAD NEWS FOODS

There is little doubt that our modern diet is the major reason for an epidemic increase in heart disease. Cultures with the lowest rate of cardiovascular disease, from Mediterranean countries to Japan, have a higher intake of vegetables and fish and a lower intake of meat. There is little doubt that the more meat you eat, the higher the risk.

WHY VEGETARIANS ARE HEALTHIER

One study looked at the meat consumption habits of 25,153 Californian Seventh Day Adventists and recorded their incidence of heart attacks over 20 years.[79] The results clearly showed a link between the amount of meat consumed and the risk of a heart attack. For 45- to 64-year-old men, those who ate meat had three times the risk of those who didn't. This finding was confirmed in a recent study by researchers at London's Department of Public Health and Policy at the London School of Hygiene and Tropical Medicine.[80] They investigated the dietary habits of over 6000 vegetarians, compared to 5000 meat eaters. Again, they found almost double the risk of a heart attack in the meat-eaters.

Whether the increased risk is due to the high saturated fat, cholesterol or other factors in meat isn't really known. There is also an association between an increased risk of heart attacks and high consumption of dairy products (milk and cheese) and eggs, although the risk is lower than that of meat. Interestingly, high dairy consumption is strongly correlated with increased risk of a stroke, while meat is more closely linked to heart attacks. In any event, the general advice is to cut back on meat and high-fat dairy produce and limit eggs, especially if fried.

SWITCH FROM MEAT TO FISH AND TOFU

Probably the best diet for the heart is a meat-free, dairy-free diet, with plenty of vegetable protein, especially tofu, and some fish. This is remarkably close to the traditional Asian diet, and may explain why Japanese people eating such a diet have one third the rate of cardiovascular disease of British people. While the benefits of eating carnivorous fish (salmon, tuna, herring, mackerel) are well known, it now appears that tofu, which is the curd of the soya bean, has its own healing properties and may be a major reason for the longer life experienced by Asians.

A review of the beneficial effects of soya confirm that it reduces cholesterol and triglycerides and raises the beneficial HDLs.[81] Italian researchers working at the University of Milan found that switching from meat to soya bean protein resulted in a 21 per cent drop in cholesterol levels, a 15 per cent drop in triglycerides and an increase in HDL in only three weeks. What's more, the beneficial effects of eating soya products were even witnessed in those eating a high-cholesterol diet. Soya beans are relatively high in phospholipids which help to escort unwanted cholesterol out of the arteries and stop too much entering in the first place. This may be partly why soya produce has a beneficial effect on cholesterol levels.

One way to increase your intake of these phospholipids is to add a tablespoonful of lecithin granules (derived from soya and available in healthfood shops) to your cereal in the morning.

This has remarkably powerful cholesterol- and triglyceride-lowering effects. In one study, cholesterol readings dropped by 31 per cent, and triglycerides by 30 per cent, while HDL went up and LDL went down.[82] All this in only four weeks.

There are many easy ways to add soya produce to your diet. Soya milk is a good substitute for milk on cereals or in drinks. Tofu comes in many forms – marinated tofu pieces, smoked tofu, braised tofu, or plain tofu (hard or soft). These can all be used in steam-fry Thai or Chinese-style dishes, much like pieces of chicken in a casserole or curry. You can even have a tofu steak, by grilling smoked tofu and putting barbecue sauce on it. Harder tofus are best for this kind of dish, while soft tofu can be added to soups or desserts instead of cream for a creamier texture.

SUGAR AND YOUR HEART

The association between high sugar, refined carbohydrate and an increased risk of cardiovascular disease is well established. In both animals and man a high intake of sugar raises triglycerides, cholesterol and insulin levels.[83] In Chapter 8, we learnt how a diet high in refined carbohydrate and sugar can lead to raised blood sugar and insulin levels, both of which have a direct effect on the health of the arteries, thus increasing the risk of cardiovascular disease.

When blood sugar levels rise, the excess glucose in the arteries immediately starts to damage proteins found in the arteries and in the lipoprotein cholesterol carriers.[84] In this way, sugar is a powerful oxidant. And it is probably through this process, more than any other, that excess sugar intake is strongly linked to increased risk of cardiovascular disease.

The average annual intake of sugar per person is 60kg (120lb). Most of this is hidden in foods. For example, several leading brands of cereal can contain as many as five different kinds of sugar (sucrose, glucose, maltose, glucose syrup,

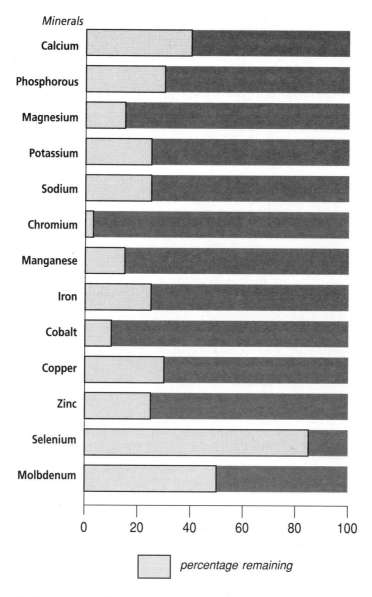

Minerals

percentage remaining

Fig 14 – Refined flour – which minerals are lost?

brown sugar and honey). If you see any of these listed on any product, you'd be better off choosing an unsweetened alternative and adding fruit.

SWITCH TO COMPLEX CARBOHYDRATES AND FRUIT

It is also best to avoid highly refined foods – those that are not in their whole, natural state. Sugar, white flour and white rice are all refined foods. Instead, choose wholemeal flour, brown rice and other whole foods such as beans, lentils, nuts and seeds. The chart on page 111 shows just what you lose in the way of life-supporting nutrients when you eat refined flour.

Oats sweetened with fresh fruit are a fine example of a wholefood dish. Oats are particularly beneficial because the fibre they contain actually helps to eliminate excess cholesterol from the body, which is why people who regularly eat oats have lower cholesterol levels.[85] Barley is also beneficial; so whole grains are definitely on the good list as far as cardiovascular health is concerned. Fresh fruits (especially apples and pears) contain fructose, a kind of sugar that the body cannot use immediately – the liver first has to convert it into glucose. This slows down its effect on raising blood sugar levels, making it easier for the body to keep them even.

So a breakfast consisting of oat flakes (as in porridge oats), a heaped tablespoon of ground seeds, chopped apple and soya milk is an excellent way to minimise your risk of heart disease, as every ingredient has beneficial properties.

THE FACTS ABOUT STIMULANTS

A scientific debate has been brewing for some years on the link between coffee and heart disease. Many studies have shown an increased risk in relation to increasing coffee consumption. For example, a study from Milan's Institute of Research and

Pharmacology found that those who drank five or more cups of coffee per day doubled their risk.[86] Other studies show increased cholesterol and LDL, lowered HDL[87] and raised blood pressure with regular coffee consumption.[88] On the other hand, there are plenty of studies that don't confirm this association. So why the confusion? It seems to depend on the type of coffee you drink. Instant, filtered or decaffeinated coffee appear to be relatively harmless, as certain chemicals that have a negative effect on cardiovascular health have been removed or substantially lowered. Boiled, unfiltered coffee, on the other hand, which is what you drink when you have a cappuccino or espresso, still contains these chemicals.

Tea has less of an association with cardiovascular risk, although very high levels of consumption are bad for the arteries due to the high tannic acid content. However tea, especially green tea which has a lower stimulant content, does also provide significant amounts of antioxidants which can be mildly protective.

The trouble is both tea and coffee contain powerful stimulants, including caffeine. A strong cup of tea contains as much caffeine as a weak cup of coffee. Chocolate and cigarettes also contain stimulants. These raise your blood sugar level because they stimulate the release of adrenal hormones which unlock stores of available glucose. So, especially for those who are insulin-resistant (see Chapter 8), this has the knock-on effect of increasing risk.

The bottom line is that addictive, regular consumption of tea and coffee is bad news, although the odd cup of unboiled coffee or, preferably, weak tea, is not a problem. Herb teas or green teas are, however, much better for you.

SALT – YOU DON'T NEED IT

While not everyone is 'salt-sensitive', the more you take in, the more potassium you need to balance it (low potassium is linked to high blood pressure). Indeed, increasing potassium in those whose diets are deficient reliably lowers blood pressure. Unfortunately the body retains salt easily and lets go of potassium. This may be due to differences in our diet since certain evolutionary processes took place: potassium was abundant and sodium was limited in the traditional hunter/gatherer diet, which was rich in fruits, vegetables, nuts and seeds. Earlier, therefore, we may have developed the ability to retain sodium, which was not so plentiful.

Although our distant ancestors may have had a much higher intake of potassium (and therefore more need to excrete it) than sodium, the modern diet has completely reversed that. Today, the average person takes in 5g of sodium and 3.5g of potassium. This is the equivalent to over 10g of salt (sodium chloride), added to food and naturally found in certain foods such as meat and cheese. The chart below shows which food groups to limit or avoid as far as salt is concerned.

How Much Sodium is There in Your Food?

Foods are listed in order of those that contain the most sodium per calorie of food. The figures in brackets are the amount of sodium in 100g, which is roughly equivalent to a cup or serving.

Shrimps	(2950mg)	Crab meat	(369mg)
Green olives	(2300mg)	Tuna fish	(339mg)
Parmesan cheese	(1862mg)	Kidney beans (canned)	(327mg)
Bacon	(1603mg)	Cream cheese	(300mg)
Ham	(1500mg)	Mussels	(286mg)
Sardines	(650mg)	Beef liver	(184mg)
Cheddar cheese	(622mg)	Egg	(138 mg)
Low-fat milk	(549mg)	Salmon	(116mg)
Cottage cheese	(405mg)	Cod	(109mg)
Whole milk	(371mg)		

There's no need to add salt to food (I haven't for 20 years), as even vegetables contain small amounts, but those who are deficient in the mineral zinc are less able to taste foods. This encourages them to add salt, which enhances flavour, and eat stronger-tasting foods such as meat and cheese. Zinc-deficiency tends to increase with age which may explain why older people eat more cheese and meat and fewer vegetables.

Not All Salt is the Same

Not all salt is bad for you. Traditional salt is simple sodium chloride. Sea salt contains other minerals, but is still predominantly sodium. Low-sodium Iceland salt, on the other hand, has a 60 per cent reduced sodium content, plus potassium and magnesium. In fact there's more potassium (21 per cent) than sodium (16 per cent), plus a small amount of magnesium (2 per cent). A research study carried out on a hundred men in Rotterdam, Holland, gave them either regular salt or the reduced sodium Iceland salt over 24 weeks.[89] The result was a significant reduction in blood pressure in those using low-sodium salt. This is a real alternative for salt addicts, although it would be better to try to get out of the habit of eating it.

ALCOHOL – IS IT GOOD FOR THE HEART?

One consistent plus for alcohol taken in moderation is the well-established finding that it increases HDL cholesterol. This is the type of cholesterol carrier that helps remove unwanted cholesterol from the arteries and is associated with lower risk. This positive effect results from drinking both beer and wine and seems to relate more to the quantity drunk than the type of drink. (Red wine in particular, may confer additional cardiovascular benefit by virtue of being high in proanthocyanidins, the antioxidants found in grapes and berries.) However, not all alcohol's effects on fats are positive: it also blocks the conversion of essential fats to their active compounds, which means the body cannot use them in cell membranes or for making prostaglandins.

Although red wine provides antioxidants, the more alcohol you consume the more antioxidants you actually need because of a complex detoxification process in the liver that requires a good supply of antioxidant nutrients, especially vitamin C. Yet, even before alcohol gets to the liver, it has negative effects in the gut where it acts as an intestinal irritant.

All in all, it is unlikely that alcohol confers any significant benefit on the cardiovascular system. While up to one small glass of red wine a day doesn't appear to increase risk, two or more alcoholic drinks a day do. An ideal intake may be less than four drinks a week.

....

CHAPTER 19

GOOD NEWS ABOUT GARLIC

For thousands of years people have been aware of the beneficial properties of garlic. The slaves who constructed the pyramids of Egypt were given garlic cloves daily to sustain their strength, as were Roman soldiers. Back in 1958, Louis Pasteur confirmed that garlic had anti-bacterial effects and, before the days of more specific antibiotics, garlic was used to treat infection. Garlic contains around 200 biologically active compounds, many of which can counteract the effects of some diseases, including heart disease.

Garlic is rich in sulphur-containing amino acids (constituents of protein) which act as antioxidants. Its beneficial effects for cardiovascular health include lowering cholesterol, protecting cholesterol from oxidation, protecting against blood clots and reducing the risk of a heart attack.[90]

GARLIC AND CHOLESTEROL

Even one clove of garlic a day can reduce a high cholesterol reading by 9 per cent, according to a review of numerous studies, made by Stephen Warshafsky at New York Medical School.[91] A report from the Royal College of Physicians in London confirmed these findings, showing an average cholesterol reduction of 12 per cent from taking garlic supplements.[92] As well as lowering cholesterol, garlic helps to protect cholesterol from oxidation. In one study by William Harris, at the University of Kansas Medical Center, patients were given six capsules containing 100mg of garlic powder for two weeks.[93] This dose reduced the oxidation of LDL cholesterol by one-third.

Garlic also thins the blood, preventing the arteries clogging up due to the formation of blood clots. The garlic does this by stopping platelets in the blood from sticking to each other. According to Eric Block, Professor of Chemistry at the State University of New York, this is probably due to a chemical within garlic called 'ajoene'. Once isolated, this compound has anti-clotting effects equivalent to those of whole garlic. Not all garlic extracts contain significant amounts of ajoene, so one of the surest ways to get all the benefits of garlic is to eat the actual clove. Three raw cloves a day will reduce clotting by about 20 per cent – the only trouble is that no one will come near you! Interestingly, cooked garlic works just as well, if not better, for reducing clotting.

GARLIC AGAINST HEART ATTACKS

Even more encouraging are the findings that garlic reduces your risk of a heart attack, even if you've already had one. A three-year study by Dr Arun Bordia at Tagore Medical College in India divided over 400 patients who had already suffered heart attacks into two groups. One group was given garlic supplements (equal to six to ten cloves per day) – they suffered fewer heart attacks and had significantly lower cholesterol counts than those who did not take garlic. After decades of research into garlic, cardiologist Dr Bordia is convinced that garlic has an important role to play in maintaining the health of the cardiovascular system.[94]

Given the known benefits of both fish oils and garlic, one wonders what their combined effect would be. A recent research trial reported that the combination of a garlic concentrate (900mg a day) and fish oil resulted in a substantial reduction in cholesterol, LDL cholesterol and blood fat levels.[95]

HOW MUCH GARLIC AND WHAT KIND?

Most studies have found benefit from taking anything from one to three cloves of garlic a day. While this dietary addition is clearly beneficial, not everyone is keen on the idea. For this reason, garlic is available as powder in capsules, or as an oil. You can even buy deodorised garlic. But do these supplements work as well as the real stuff? Of the hundreds of active chemicals in garlic, two have been proven to be especially beneficial – allicin and ajoene. If you take capsules rather than cloves of garlic, do check that these two vital ingredients haven't been processed out. If the details are not stated on the label call the manufacturer and ask them.

CHAPTER 20

....

CO-ENZYME Q AND YOUR HEART

Another nutrient, Co-Enzyme Q10, shows an extraordinary ability to help patients with heart disease and other diseases in which energy production within body cells is not efficient. So astonishing are the properties of this nutrient that no less than 12 million people in Japan supplement their diets with Co-Q. In Kiev a research institute was set up solely to study the effects of this remarkable nutrient.

Co-Q was first isolated 40 years ago in Britain, by a group of scientists working in Liverpool, and was identified as a critical component in the production of energy within cells. It has recently been discovered that Co-Q is present in foods, that levels decline with age, and that cellular levels rise when supplements are taken; these discoveries have led many scientists to consider Co-Q as an undiscovered vitamin. Technically, however, Co-Q cannot be classified as a vitamin since it can be made by the body, although not in sufficient amounts for optimum health and energy. It is therefore a semi-essential nutrient – in other words, some Co-Q must be consumed in the diet.

CO-Q AND ENERGY PRODUCTION IN CELLS

In the final, and most significant stage in energy production, when hydrogen reacts with oxygen, the latent energy in food is literally released as tiny charged particles, called electrons. These are highly reactive and need to be handled carefully. They are like nuclear fuel – a very powerful, but potentially very dangerous energy source.

So dangerous are these spare electrons that, if not properly controlled, they are thought to be the initiating factor in damaging artery walls, heralding the beginning of heart disease or even making some cells cancerous. The damage they cause to healthy cells is largely what the ageing process is all about. The more damaged cells we have, the older we are biochemically. Compounds that contain spare electrons act as oxidants. They are created both during normal energy metabolism, and also by smoking, eating fried food, breathing in pollution, and being exposed to radiation from the sun.

Co-Q has two key roles to play in handling these volatile electrons. It controls the flow of oxygen, making the production of energy extremely efficient, and prevents damage caused by spare electrons. It is therefore a key antioxidant in the body. According to Dr Folkers, Director of the Institute for Biomedical Research at Austin University in Texas, once body levels of Co-Q drop below 25 per cent of normal, disease may ensue.

In the last decade, well over a hundred research trials using Co-Q have been conducted in the USA and Japan with some astonishing results. Since it has such a critical part to play in the energy production of every single cell, Co-Q's use in promoting health is far-reaching and perhaps best illustrated by recent trials on heart disease patients.

CO-Q AND CARDIOVASCULAR DISEASE

A six-year study at the University of Texas involved people with congestive heart failure, a condition in which the heart, the largest muscle in the human body, becomes progressively weaker. Results showed that 75 per cent of those on Co-Q survived three years, compared to 25 per cent on conventional medication.[96] In no less than 20 properly controlled studies published in the last two years, Co-Q has repeatedly demonstrated a remarkable ability to improve heart function and has now become the treatment of choice in Japan. In a combined trial by the University of Austin, Texas, and the Centre for Adult Diseases in Osaka, Japan, 52 patients with high blood pressure were treated either with Co-Q or dummy tablets.[97] There was an 11 per cent decrease in blood pressure for those on Co-Q, compared to a 2 per cent decrease for those on dummy tablets.

Angina is a common condition in which sufferers experience pain in the heart region when they exert themselves. It is usually caused by blockages in the tiny arteries that feed the heart muscle cells with oxygen. Since Co-Q helps all muscle cells to become more efficient, this magical nutrient has also been investigated as a natural treatment for angina. In one study at Hamamatsu University in Japan, angina patients treated with Co-Q were able to increase their tolerance of exercise and had less frequent angina attacks.[98] After only four weeks on Co-Q, other medication could be halved.

Co-Q, at a daily dose of 90mg, has also been shown to reduce oxidation damage in the arteries, thereby protecting fats in the blood (such as LDL cholesterol) from becoming damaged and contributing to arterial blockages.[99]

While a diet containing fish, nuts and seeds provides significant amounts of Co-Q, the therapeutic effects are rarely seen below an intake of 90mg a day which can only be achieved with supplementation. Many supplements contain 30mg, making it necessary to take three tablets a day. Co-Q is also much better absorbed in an oil-based form so it is best to choose supplements that state this on the label.[100]

Which foods are Rich in Co-Enzyme Q10?

Food	Amount (mg per 100g)	Food	Amount (mg per 100g)
Meat		*Beans*	
Beef	3.1	Green beans	0.58
Pork	2.4–4.1	Soya beans	0.29
Chicken	2.1	Aduki beans	0.22
Fish		*Nuts and seeds*	
Sardines	6.4	Peanuts	2.7
Mackerel	4.3	Sesame seeds	2.3
Flat fish	0.5	Walnuts	1.9
Grains		*Vegetables*	
Rice bran	0.54	Spinach	1
Rice	–	Broccoli	0.8
Wheatgerm	0.35	Peppers	0.3
Wheatflour	–	Carrots	0.2
Millet	0.15	*Oils*	
Buckwheat	0.13	Soya oil	9.2

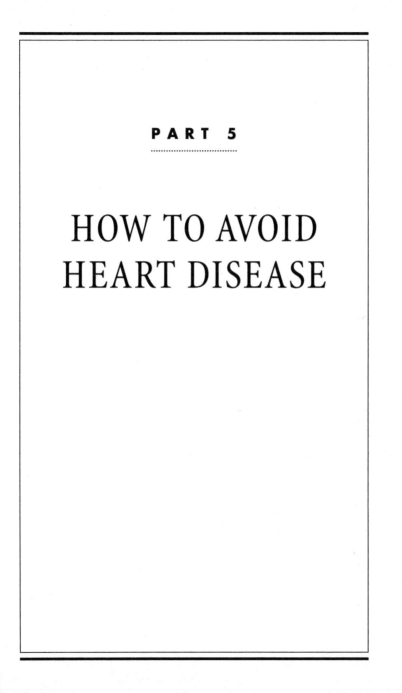

PART 5

HOW TO AVOID
HEART DISEASE

CHAPTER 21

THE IDEAL DIET

O n the basis of all the evidence presented in this book, it is now clear what you need to eat, drink and avoid to maximise your health and minimise your risk of cardiovascular disease. This chapter spells it out in two ways. First, there's a list of foods and drinks to increase and to decrease, giving you ideal targets to aim at, and practical suggestions about which foods to eat. These suggestions are ideal for preventing and reversing cardiovascular disease. Depending on your current eating habits and tastes, you may find changes hard to achieve at first. But, once you start making realistic steps towards your goal, your tastes will gradually change and you will start to feel better.

At the end of the chapter there's a typical day's menu that incorporates all the beneficial foods showing how you can enjoy your food *and* eat yourself to health.

There are many, many different dishes you can concoct using foods that promote cardiovascular health, rather than reduce it. Of all the foods and eating principles we've discussed, probably the most important ones are: to eat five servings of fruits and vegetables a day; cut back on meat – choosing fish or soya products instead; eat some seeds or their oils every day; and avoid frying. You can 'steam-fry' by adding a watery sauce to a pan full of, say vegetables and tofu, putting the lid on tight and steaming in the sauce.

The Healthy Heart Plan

Foods to Increase

- Fruit and vegetables – five servings every day
- Carnivorous fish – three times a week
- Seeds – a heaped tablespoon every day
- Cold-pressed seed oils – for salads and spreads
- Tofu – three times a week
- Garlic – a clove or two every day

Foods to Decrease

- Alcohol – no more than 4 units a week
- Meat – stick to fish three times a week and chicken once, if at all
- Eggs – no more than three a week, free-range, not fried
- Dairy products – minimal, substitute soya milk
- Tea – no more than two cups a day
- Coffee – no more than one cup a day (not both tea and coffee in the same day)
- Sugar in its many disguises – don't add it and avoid foods with added sugar
- Salt – none or small amount of low-sodium salt

A Typical Healthy Heart Menu

BREAKFAST
1 cup of oat flakes (porridge oats)
1 heaped tablespoon of ground seeds (sesame, sunflower, pumpkin and flax)
1 tablespoon of lecithin granules
A chopped organic apple or pear
1 cup of soya milk

MID-MORNING SNACK
An organic apple or pear, plus 10 almonds

LUNCH
Baked Potato with Tuna and Corn
or
Marinated or Smoked Tofu, Tahini and
Watercress Rye Sandwich
or
Rainbow Root Salad
or
Shiitake Mushrooms, Tofu and Vegetables
Carrot Soup in the Raw and Oatcakes

MID-AFTERNOON SNACK
An organic apple or pear and 10 almonds

DINNER
Vegetable Steam-Fry followed by Berry (soya) Ice-cream
or
Almond Mackerel with New Potatoes and Lemon Kale
or
Poached Salmon with Mashed Sweet Potato and Brussels
Sprouts in a Hummus and Mushroom Sauce

(The recipes for all these dishes are taken from my book
100% Health).

....

CHAPTER 22

SUPPLEMENTARY BENEFIT

Whatever your opinions about taking supplements, the truth is that supplementing a combination of the right nutrients is more effective in the longer term than taking drugs designed to lower blood pressure or reduce the risk of a heart attack or stroke. Supplements deal with the cause of the problem, rather than the symptoms. The nutrients discussed in this book promote cardiovascular health when taken in the doses suggested. Even a well-balanced diet is unlikely to provide anywhere near these levels. I take supplements every day because I feel better, have seen them literally save people's lives, want to live a long and healthy life, and know that they can only do me good.

The ideal levels vary from person to person and, for maximum cardiovascular health, I recommend you take the quantities shown in the chart overleaf, as well as eating as nutritious a diet as you can. I have listed the ideal levels for basic prevention and the range for therapeutic use for those at risk. The therapeutic levels are best taken with the advice and support of your doctor or a nutrition consultant. A directory of nutrition consultants is available from the Institute for Optimum Nutrition (see page 146).

Ideal Supplementary Nutrient intake for a Healthy Heart

Nutrient	For Basic Prevention	For Those at Risk
Vitamins		
Vitamin A	*20,000iu*	
as retinol	*10,000iu*	
as beta-carotene	*10,000iu*	
Vitamin C	*1000mg*	*2000–10,000mg*
Vitamin D	400iu	
Vitamin E	*150mg (200iu)*	*400mg (500iu)*
B1 (Thiamine)	25mg	
B2 (Riboflavin)	25mg	
B3 (Niacin)	*25mg*	*500mg*
B5 (Pantothenic acid)	25 mg	
B6 (Pyridoxine)	*25mg*	*50mg*
B12	10mcg	
Folic acid	*100mcg*	*400mcg*
Biotin	50mcg	
Minerals		
Calcium	*350mg*	*800mg*
Magnesium	*200mg*	*500mg*
Zinc	15mg	25mg
Iron	10mg	
Manganese	5mg	10mg
Chromium	50mcg	100mcg
Selenium	*100mcg*	*200mcg*
Amino Acids		
Lysine	*500mg*	*3000mg*
Reduced glutathione	50mg	100mg
or N-acetyl cysteine	500mg	1000mg
Essential Fats		
EPA	*300mg*	*1000mg+*
GLA	150mg	250mg
Other		
Co-enzyme Q10	*30mg*	*90mg*

The most important nutrients are printed in *italic*.

In practical terms, the easiest way to achieve these levels is to take:

- A good all-round multivitamin and multimineral plus extra vitamin C

- An antioxidant complex

- Plus 'extras' if your risk is high

The chart overleaf shows the extra levels to supplement for basic prevention, and for those at risk (high blood pressure or a history of cardiovascular disease), in addition to a good all-round multivitamin, vitamin C and an antioxidant complex.

	Antioxidant	Multivitamin plus C	Suggested 'extras' for basic protection	Suggested 'extras' for those at risk
Vitamin A as retinol	5000iu (1.5mgRE)	5000iu (1.5mgRE)		
Vitamin A as beta-carotene	5000iu(1.5mgRE)	5000iu (1.5mgRE)		
Vitamin C	500mg	500mg		2000–10,000mg
Vitamin E	50mg	100mg		250mg (400iu)
Vitamin D		400iu		
Vitamin B1 (Thiamine)		25mg		
Vitamin B2 (Riboflavin)		25mg		
Vitamin B3 (Niacin)		50mg		500mg
Vitamin B5 (Pantothenic Acid)		50mg		
Vitamin B6 (Pyridoxine)		50mg		
Vitamin B12		10mcg		
Folic acid		100mcg		300mcg
Biotin		50mcg		
Lysine			500mg	2500mg
Reduced glutathione			50mg	100mg
or N-acetyl cysteine			or 500mg	1000mg
Proanthocyanidins (e.g. bilberry, grape seed)	100mg			
Pycnogenol (from pine)	5mg			
Silymarin (from milk thistle)	100mg			
Calcium		350mg		450mg
Magnesium		200mg		300mg
Chromium		50mcg		50mcg
Selenium	50mcg	50mcg		100mcg
Zinc	5mg	10mg		10mg
Manganese	2mg	3mg		5mg
Iron		10mg		
EPA			300mg	1000mg
GLA			150mg	250mg
Co-enzyme Q10			30mg	90mg

A typical supplement programme designed to minimise cardiovascular risk may be as follows:

	For Prevention	For Those at Risk
Multivitamin/mineral	2 (normal daily dose)	4
Antioxidant complex	2 (normal daily dose)	
Vitamin C 1000mg	1	4
Vitamin E 400iu (250mg)		1
Vitamin B3 (Niacin) 250mg		2
Folic acid 400mcg		1
Lysine 500/1000mg	1	2
N-acetyl cysteine 1000mg		1
Multimineral		2
EPA fish oil 300mg	1	3
GLA 150/250mg	1	1
Co-enzyme Q10 30/90mg	1	1

Take your supplements with food, unless otherwise stated. Many vitamins help to boost your energy levels and so are best taken with breakfast or lunch. Calcium and magnesium have a calming effect and are best taken with dinner, especially if you have difficulty getting to sleep. Most important of all, stick to your supplement programme every day. It can take three months before you notice the beneficial effects. They are worth waiting for.

CHAPTER 23

LIFESTYLE CHANGES

All you need to do (along with a change in diet plus supplements), to minimise your risk of heart disease, is make four simple lifestyle changes. These lifestyle changes are, of course, highly beneficial in many other ways – generally improving your sense of well-being and vitality.

Keep Fit Not Fat

Even 30 minutes a week of aerobic exercise (raising your pulse by 80 per cent) makes a difference to the fitness of your cardiovascular system. More strengthens your heart and arteries. It also helps to boost your metabolic rate and keep you slim. Being overweight puts an extra strain on your heart and arteries. The best forms of exercise are brisk walking, hill-walking, jogging, swimming, cycling or aerobics. Find a sport you enjoy and play it once a week. Regular exercise once a week might not seem like much to start with but it really makes a difference in the long run. Aim for at least half an hour three times a week or 15 minutes a day.

One of my favourite forms of exercise for tuning up the cardiovascular system is Psychocalisthenics, developed by Oscar Ichazo of the Arica Institute in New York. The word means strength (*sthenia*) and beauty (*cali*) through the breath (*psyche*); it involves a unique series of 22 exercises which develop strength, suppleness and stamina, oxygenating the whole body. Psychocalisthenics is suitable for anyone – young or old. It takes a day to learn and, once learnt, you can do it in 15 minutes, accompanied by a tape or video. Psychocalisthenics classes take place all over the UK and US. (For details, see Useful Addresses on page 146.)

Too much exercise, on the other hand, can elevate levels of the stress hormone cortisol and is not recommended if you are stressed out. On the other hand, Psychocalisthenics, yoga, Tai Chi or walking for half an hour can help to re-balance stress hormones. So, too, can meditation.

Avoid Prolonged Stress

Keep cool. Stress raises your blood pressure by causing blood vessels to constrict and the heart to beat faster. Notice your personal signs of tension (clenched fists, tight shoulders, nail biting, shallow breathing, etc) and observe what circumstances make you react stressfully. Notice how you react. Do you drink more, eat more, become hyperactive, get cross? Once you know what causes you stress and how you react, you're more than halfway there. Then you have two options. Realise that it doesn't serve you to react stressfully in these situations. Or, if you are continually in a situation that causes you stress, get out of the situation if you can. You'll handle stress much better if you avoid excessive use of stimulants such as tea, coffee, chocolate and cigarettes.

Stop Smoking

Smoking triggers cell damage, starves healthy cells of oxygen, thickens the blood and raises your blood pressure. Of the deaths caused by smoking, twice as many are due to diseases of the heart and arteries as are due to lung cancer. The less you smoke, the better. But, best of all, stop smoking.

Check Your Blood Pressure and Blood Fats

Check your blood pressure and your blood levels of cholesterol, triglycerides, LDLs and HDLs at least every three years
– your doctor can do these tests for you. The older you are,
the more frequently you should have checks. If you have any
risk at all, be it symptoms, high blood pressure or a previous
cardiovascular event (such as a stroke or heart attack), you
should also check your lipoprotein (a) and homocysteine levels. If your doctor doesn't know about these important risk
factors, find your nearest nutrition consultant by calling the
Institute for Optimum Nutrition (see page 146) who can also
run all these tests for you. Make sure you keep a copy of the
results so you can compare your levels to those given in this
book. When your blood fats and your blood pressure are low
your risk is minimal.

CHAPTER 24

MAXIMISING RECOVERY

If you've had a heart attack or stroke and want to maximise your recovery there's plenty that you can do. Most return of function takes place in the first six months afterwards, so that is the time to make sure your body has maximum nutritional support. Needless to say, everything recommended in previous chapters for a person 'at risk' applies to you, and there's more.

USING OXYGEN EFFICIENTLY

Strokes and heart attacks often temporarily starve areas of tissue (cells) of oxygen, possibly resulting in reduced or complete lack of circulation. So, what can you do to get nutrients, especially oxygen, through? The answer is to increase your intake of vitamin E, Co-Enzyme Q10, vitamin C and other antioxidants. These nutrients will maximise the delivery to and use of oxygen in recovering cells. So, increase your daily intake from supplements to:

- Co-Enzyme Q10   180mg

- Vitamin E   800mg (1000iu)

- Vitamin C   6000mg

- Antioxidant formula   3 rather than 2 a day

REBUILDING HEALTHY CELLS

The body is remarkably good at regenerating its cells – and some important nutrients help this process. Cells are basically containers that keep the watery 'outside' out and the nutrients they need in. The membrane that allows this controlled separation is made from phospholipids and fatty acids. By increasing your intake of these phospholipids, especially phosphatidyl serine (PS), you can maximise repair of cells, particularly in the nervous system. The results can be quite spectacular.

PS is derived from lecithin, which is itself derived from soya beans. Lecithin especially enriched with PS is also rich in phosphatidyl choline (PC) which helps make the key memory neurotransmitter acetylcholine. Together, these nutrients help to maximise the recovery of cells, particularly of the nervous system. You may be able to find lecithin granules enriched with PS, in which case you can add this to your cereal. Otherwise, take an actual supplement.

Another key membrane-building nutrient is an amino acid called glutamine. This helps rebuild muscle after injury or surgery and is the most abundant amino acid in the cerebrospinal fluid. Although untested, logic dictates that glutamine may help recovery after a stroke or heart attack. The easiest and cheapest way to supplement glutamine is to take it as a powder. As it is tasteless, it can be dissolved in water or juice or put on your morning cereal.

So, if you've had a stroke or heart attack, you may benefit from adding, for the first few months afterwards, the following supplements:

- Phosphatidyl serine   300mg (600mg for first two weeks)
- Glutamine   3000mg (6000mg for first two weeks)

Half these levels is an optional maintenance dose, once maximum recovery has been achieved. Essential fatty acids are also vital, although there's no need to supplement above the level for 'those at risk' shown on page 130.

Drug–nutrient interactions

After a cardiovascular event the chances are that you will be prescribed a combination of drugs. Since some of these drugs, such as aspirin, aim to thin the blood, you have to be careful about adding nutrients which achieve the same effect in case you over-thin the blood. The nutrients which do this are the fish oil EPA (strong effect), vitamin E and B3 (mild effect). If you are taking all these in therapeutic doses it is unlikely that you will need aspirin; however that is for you to decide in discussion with your doctor.

While I have tried to make cardiovascular health simple to understand, the truth is that it is a complex business. There are many different nutrients to consider and no programme is perfect for everyone. Therefore, I strongly advise you to contact a nutrition consultant who can guide you through the maze and advise you on *your* specific needs. Most of all, I wish you good luck, not only in maximising your recovery, but also in finding a level of health and well-being beyond that which you have previously experienced.

REFERENCES

The references listed here relate to the main studies referred to, and numbered, in the text. Those readers who wish to dig deeper are advised to access the scientific literature held on file at the Institute for Optimum Nutrition, who can carry out literature and library searches on any topic of interest.

1. Holford, P., *Optimum Nutrition*, p 52, ION Press (1992).

2. Cannon, M. et al, 'The effect of combined micronutrient supplementation on blood pressure' (1990), paper held by ION library, available from ION, London.

3. Colgan, M., Institute of Nutritional Science, unpublished material held in ION library.

4. Reported at the International Congress of Nutrition in Kyoto, Japan, 1975, by Dr R. Alfin-Slater.

5. Passwater, R., *Supernutrition for a Healthy Heart*, p 67, Thorsons/Harper-Collins (1977).

6. Hirshowitz, B. et al, '35 Eggs Per Day in the Treatment of Severe Burns', *Br. J. Plast Surg.*, vol 28: 3, pp 85–8 (1975).

7. Herbert, P., *Medical World News* (February 1977).

8. 'Report of the Advisory Panel of the Committee on Medical Aspects of Food Policy on Diet in Relation to Cardiovascular and Cerebrovascular Disease, Diet and Coronary Heart Disease', London (1974).

9. Jolliffe research referred to in (5) above.

10. De Oliviera e Silva et al, *Am. J. Clin. Nutr.*, vol 64:5 pp 712–7 (1996).

11. Russell, R., 'Soy protein and nutrition', *JAMA*, vol 277:23 pp 1876–8 (1997).

12. Grundy, S. et al, 'Influence of nicotinic acid on metabolism of cholesterol and triglycerides in man', *J. Lipid Res.* vol 22, pp 24–36 (1981).

13. Hoeg, J. et al, 'Special communication: an approach to the management of hyperlipoproteinemia', *Metabolism*, vol 34:11, pp 1073–7 (1985).

14. O'Connor, P., Rush, W. et al, 'Relative effectiveness of niacin and lovastatin for treatment of dyslipidemias in a health maintenance organization', *J. Fam. Pract.* vol 44:5 pp 462–7 (May 1997).

15. Illingworth, D., Stein, E. et al, 'Comparative effects of lovastatin and niacin in primary hypercholesterolemia. A prospective trial,' *Arch. Intern. Med.*, vol 154:14, pp 1586–95 (25 July 1994).

16. Gardner, S., Schneider, E. et al., 'Combination therapy with low-dose lovastatin and niacin is as effective as higher dose lovastatin', *Pharmacotherapy*, vol 16:3, pp 419–23 (May 1996).

17. Vega, G., Grundy, S., 'Lipoprotein responses to treatment with lovastatin, gemfibrozil and nicotinic acid in normolipidemic patients with hypoalphalipoprotein,' *Arch. Intern. Med.*, vol 154:1, pp 73–82 (10 Jan. 1994).

18. Ueshima, H. et al., *Prevent. Med.*, vol 8:1, pp 104–5 (1979).

19. *New Scientist* (29 April 1995) p 10.

20. David Freedman, 'Centers for Disease Control,' in *Optimum Nutrition*, vol 8:2, pp 8–9 (1995).

21. Wald, N.J., 'Apolipoproteins and ischaemic heart disease,' *Lancet* (8 Jan. 1994). 'Apolipoproteins and ischaemic heart disease,' *Journal Royal Soc. of Health* (April 1994). *Science* (14 August 1993).

22. Sinclair, H., *Drugs Affecting Lipid Metabolism*, ARIPS Press, distributor for Elsevier Horth-Holland Inc. Biomedical Press, Arlington, VA (1980).

23. Hirai, A. et al, *Lancet*, pp 1132–3 (22 Nov 1980).

24. Kato, H. et al, *Am. J. of Epidemiology 97*, vol 6:73, pp 372–85.

25. Kromhout, D., *Proc. of the Nutr. Soc.*, vol 52, pp 437–9.

26. Dolecek, T. et al, *World Rev. of Nutr. and Dietetics*, vol 66, pp 205–16 (MRFIT).

27. Leng et al, *Prostaglandins Leukot Essent Fatty Acids (Scotland)*, vol 51:2, pp 101–8 (Aug 1994).

28. Burr, M. et al, *Lancet*, vol 2, pp 757–61 (1989).

29. Stensvold, I. et al, 'Non-pasting serum triglyceride concentration and mortality from coronary heart disease and any cause in middle-aged Norwegian women,' *BMJ*, vol 307 (6915) pp 1318–22 (20 November 1993).

30. Pyzh, M.V. et al, *Kardiologiia*, vol 33:10, pp 46–50, 5–6 (1993) and Kobayashi, S. et al, *Lancet*, p 197 (25 July 1981).

31. Sanders, T. and Younger, K., *Brit. J. Nutr.*, vol 45, p 613 (1981).

32. Saynor, R. and Verel, D., *IRCS Med. Sci.*, vol 8, p 378–9 (1980). Saynor, R. and Verel, D., *Throm. Haem.*, vol 46:91, p 65 (1981) and personal communication.

33. Tamari, G., *Townsend Newsletter for Doctors* (May 1995).

34. McVeigh, G.E. et al, *Arterioscler. Thromb.*, vol 14:9, p 1425–9 (1994).

35. Mori, T., *Metabolism*, vol 40, pp 241–6 (1991). Danno K. et al, *Arch. Dermatol. Res.*, vol 285:7, pp 432–5 (1993).

36. 'Renaud and the mystery of the Cretan diet,' *Elan* (24 June 1994).

37. Rath, M. et al. 'A unified theory of human cardiovascular disease leading the way to the abolition of this disease as a cause of human mortality,' *J. Ortho. Med.*, vol 7:1, pp 5–12 (1992).

38. Rath, M. and Pauling, Linus, 'Hypothesis: Lipoprotein (a) is a surrogate for ascorbate,' *Proc. Natl. Acad. Sci. USA*, vol 87, pp 6204–7 (August 1990).

39. Lawn R., 'Lipoprotein (a) in heart disease,' *Scientific American*, pp 26–32 (June 1992).

40. Patent Application Ser. No. 07/533.129, 'Prevention and treatment of occlusive cardiovascular disease with ascorbate and substances that inhibit the binding of lipoprotein (a),' (Filed 1990).

41. Gardner, S., Schneider, E. et al., see (16) above.

42. Holmes, D., 'An answer to angina,' *Holistic Health* vol 49, pp 20–3 (1995).

43. Reaven, G., 'Role of Insulin Resistance in Human Disease,' *Diabetes*, vol 37, pp 1595–1607 (1988).

44. Broughton, D., Taylor, R., 'Deterioration of Glucose Tolerance with Age: The Role of Insulin Resistance,' *Age & Aging*, vol 20, pp 221–5 (1991).

45. Sears, Barry, *Enter The Zone*, Regan Books HarperCollins, available from ION, London (1995).

46. Gaugean, R. et al, *Am. J. Clin. Nutr.*, vol 65 (3), pp 861–70 (March 1997).

47. *Newsweek* (11 August, 1997).

48. Selhub, J. et al, 'Association between plasma homocysteine concentrations and extracranial carotid artery stenosis,' *New England Journal of Medicine*, vol 332:5, pp 286–91 (1995).

49. Graham, I. et al, 'Plasma homocysteine as a risk factor for vascular disease,' *JAMA* vol 277:22, pp 1775–81 (1997).

50. *Lancet*, vol 2 (8197), pp 720–2 (4 Oct. 1980).

51. Turlapaty, P. and Altura, B., *Science*, vol 208: pp 198–200 (11 April 1980).

52. Altura, B. and Altura, B., 'Magnesium in Cardiovascular Biology,' *Scientific American*, pp 28–36 (May/June 1995).

53. *Angiology*, vol 28 (10), pp 720–24 (Oct. 1977).

54. Altura, B. and Altura B., see (52) above.

55. Forsén, T. et al., 'Mother's weight in pregnancy and coronary heart disease in a cohort of Finnish men: follow-up study,' *BMJ*, vol 315, pp 837–40 (1997).

56. Wiley, R. et al. 'Isometric exercise training lowers resting blood pressure,' *Med. Sci. Sports Exercise*, vol 24, pp 749–54 (1992).

57. Cheraskin, E. 'Medical (not health) care costs are rising…stupid!,' *J. Adv. Med.*, vol 7:4, pp 223–30 (1994).

58. Gullette, E. et al, 'Effects of mental stress on myocardial ischemia during daily life,' *JAMA*, vol 277: 2220, pp 1521–6 (1997).

59. Patel, C. 'Trial of relaxation in reducing coronary risk: four year follow-up,' *Brit. Med. J.*, vol 290, p 1103 (1985).

60. Stephens, N. et al, 'Randomised controlled trial of vitamin E in patients with coronary disease: Cambridge Heart Antioxidant Study (CHAOS),' *Lancet*, p 347 (23 March 1996).

61. Stamper, M.J. et al, *New Engl. J. Med.*, pp 1444–9 (20 May 1993).

62. Stamper, M.J. et al, *New Engl. J. Med.*, pp 1450–5 (20 May 1993).

63. Losonczy, K.G. et al, *Am. J. Clin. Nutr.*, vol 64, pp 190–6 (1996).

64. Diaz, M., Frei, B., Vita, J. and Keaney, J., 'Antioxidants and atherosclerotic heart disease,' *New Engl. J. Med.*, vol 337:6 pp 408–14 (1997).

65. Scherak, O. and Kolarz, G., 'Vitamin E and Rheumatoid Arthritis,' *Arthritis Rheum.*, vol 34:9, pp 1205–6 (1991).

66. Jacques, P., 'Effects of vitamin C on high-density lipoprotein cholesterol and blood pressure,' *Am. J. Coll. Nutr.*, vol 11:2, pp 139–44 (1992).

67. Osilesi, O. et al, 'Blood pressure and plasma lipids during ascorbic acid supplementation in borderline hypertensive and normotensive adults,' *Nutr. Res.* vol 11, pp 405–12 (1991).

68. Block, G., 'Vitamin C, cancer and aging,' *Age*, vol 16, pp 55–8 (1993).

69. Alexander, M., Newmark, H. and Miller, R., 'Oral beta-carotene can increase the number of OKT4+ cells in human blood,' *Immunol. Lett*, vol 9, pp 221–4 (1985).

70. Heliovaara, M., Knekt, P. and Aho, K. et al, 'Serum antioxidants and risk of rheumatoid arthritis,' *Ann. Rheum*, vol 53:1 pp 51–3 (1994).

71. McCarron, D., 'Role of adequate dietary calcium intake in the prevention and management of salt-sensitive hypertension,' *Am. J. Clin. Nutr.*, vol 65:2S pp 712S–716S (1997).

Osborne, C. et al, 'Evidence for the relationship of calcium to blood pressure,' *Nutr. Rev.*, vol 54:12, pp 366–81 (1996).

Whelton, P. et al, 'Effects of oral potassium on blood pressure,' *JAMA*, vol 2777:20, pp 1624–32 (1997).

Dyckner, T., *BMJ*, vol 286, pp 1847–9 (1983).

72. Cannon, M. et al, see (2) above.

73. *The Booker Health Report*, Research by Queen Elizabeth College, University of London, Booker Health Foods (1985).

74. Osborne, C., see (71) above.

75. Whiting, S. et al., 'Adverse effects of high calcium diets in humans,' *Nutrition Reviews* vol 55:1, pp 1–9 (1997).

76. Whelton, P. see (71) above.

77. Appel, L. et al., 'A clinical trial of the effects of dietary patterns on blood pressure', *New Engl. J. Med.*, vol 336:16, pp 1117–24 (1997).

78. Chazin, S., 'Is Iron a Danger in Your Diet?' *Reader's Digest* (Dec. 1995).

79. Snowden, D. et al., 'Meat consumption and fatal ischemic heart disease,' *Preventive Medicine*, vol 13:5, pp 490–500 (1984).

80. Throgood, M. et al., 'Risk of death from cancer and ischaemic heart disease in meat,' *BMJ*, vol 308:6945, pp 1667–70 (1994).

81. Carroll, K., 'Review of clinical studies on cholesterol-lowering response to soy bean,' *J. Am. Diet. Assoc.*, vol 91, pp 820–7 (1991).

82. Kupke, D. et al., *Medwelt*, vol 38, pp 1244–7 (1987).

83. Yudkin, J., 'Sugar and disease,' *Nature*, vol 239, pp 197–9 (1972).

84. Furth, A. and Harding, J., 'Why sugar is bad for you,' *New Scientist*, pp 44–7 (23 Sept 1989).

85. Welch, R., 'Can dietary oats promote health?' *Brit. J. Biomed. Sci.*, vol 51, pp 260–70 (1994).

86. D'Avanzo, B., 'Coffee consumption and risk of acute myocardial infarction,' *Ann. Epidemiol*, vol 3:6, pp 595–604 (1993).

87. Berndt, B. et al., 'Lipoprotein metabolism and coffee intake – who is at risk?' *Z Ernahrungswiss*, vol 32:3, pp 163–75 (1993).

88. Sung, B. et al., Caffeine elevates blood pressure response to exercise in mild hypertensive men, *Am. J. Hypertens*, vol 8:12.1, pp 1184–8 (1995).

89. Geleijnse, J. et al., 'Reduction in blood pressure with a low sodium, high potassium, high magnesium salt in older subjects with mild to moderate hypertension,' *BMJ* vol 309, pp 436–40 (1994).

90. Lau, B. et al., 'Garlic and Atherosclerosis: A review,' *Nutr. Res.*, vol 3, pp 119–28 (1983).

91. Warshafsky, S., 'Effect of garlic on total serum cholesterol. A meta-analysis,' *Ann. of Int. Med.*, vol 119:7.1 pp 599–605 (1993).

92. Silagy, C., 'Garlic as a lipid lowering agent – a meta-analysis,' *J. Royal Coll. Phys.*, vol 28:1 pp 39–45 (1994).

93. Carper, Jean, *Stop Ageing Now*, p 160, HarperCollins (1995).

94. *Ibid.*, pp 161–2.

95. Adler, A. and Holub, B., 'Effect of garlic and fish oil supplementation on serum lipid and lipoprotein concentrations in hypercholesterolemic men,' *Am. J. Clin. Nutr.*, vol 65:2, pp 445–50 (1997).

96. Folkers, K. and Yamamura, Y. ed, *Biomedical and Clinical Aspects of Coenzyme Q*, Elsevier Science Publishers, BV, Amsterdam (1986).

97. See (96) above.

98. See (96) above.

99. Kaikkonen, J. et al., 'Effect of oral coenzyme Q10 supplementation on the oxidation resistance of human VLDL and LDL fraction: absorption and antioxidative properties of oil and granule-based preparations,' *Free Rad. Biol. Med.*, vol 22:7, pp 1195–1202 (1997).

Mohr, D. et al, 'Dietary supplementation with coenzyme Q10 results in higher levels of ubiquinol-10 within circulating lipoproteins and inceased resistance of human low-density lipoprotein to the initiation of lipid peroxidation,' *Biochimica et Biophysica Acta*, vol 1126, pp 247–54 (1992).

100. Kaikkonen, J., see (99) above.

USEFUL ADDRESSES

British Society for Allergy, Environmental and Nutritional Medicine
The organisation for medical doctors working with allergies (including chemical sensitivities) and nutritional problems. Full members are all doctors; associate membership and other categories exist for related professions. Holds regular meetings and supports the publication of the *Journal of Nutritional and Environmental Medicine*. For further information visit www.jnem.demon.co.uk.

Institute for Optimum Nutrition (ION)
ION runs courses from a Home Study course to a Foundation Degree in Nutritional Therapy and regularly organises lectures for health professionals and the general public. Services and facilities include a membership scheme, subscription to *Optimum Nutrition* magazine, a library and information centre, nutritional therapy clinics and a printed directory listing DipION Nutritional Therapists across the UK and overseas. For further information, write to **ION**, Avalon House, 72 Lower Mortlake Road, Richmond TW9 2JY. Tel: 020 8614 7800, or visit www.ion.ac.uk.

MetaFitness teach the excellent exercise system Psychocalisthenics, referred to in this book. For further details of nationwide classes contact: **MetaFitness**, Squires Hill House, Tilford, Surrey GU10 2AD. Tel: 01252 782661.

Nutrition Consulations
For personal referral by Patrick Holford to a nutritional therapist in your area, visit www.patrickholford.com and click on 'Advice' and then 'Find a nutritionist'. If there is no one available nearby, you can get your own personal diet and supplement programme by completing the online 100% Health Programme.

Nutritional Supplements are available from a wide variety of companies. Two companies who provide an extensive range, between them covering the speciality supplements referred to in this book are **Solgar**, available in health food shops, and **BioCare** (call 0121 433 3727 or visit www.biocare.co.uk). Connect is a combination of nutrients designed to enhance methylation and reduce homocysteine levels and is available from Biocare.

INDEX

acetylcholine 138
ajoene 118, 119
alcohol 6, 25, 70, 78, 83, 101, 104,
    115, 127
allergies 35
allicin 119
alpha-tocopherol 92
Alzheimer's disease 3, 4
amino acids 117, 138
angina 16, 34, 42, 43, 61, 101, 121
anti-nutrients 101
antioxidants 6, 25, 51, 56, 69, 78, 79,
    91, 95–8, 107, 115, 117, 121, 131,
    137
apoprotein 26, 38–9
arterial disease 35, *Fig 7*
arteries 8
    blocked 3, 14–16, 50, 56, 61, 72, 82,
        91, 122
    damaged 93, 121
    inflammation of 46, 50, 91
    in spasm 61, 62–3, *Fig 10*
arthritis 3, 4
aspirin 34–5, 42, 50, 88, 139
asthma 35
atherosclerosis 3, 11, 14–16, 25, 39, 46,
    59, 61–2, 75, 81, *Fig 3*
    reversing 41–3

beta-blockers 42, 43
beta-carotene 69, 79, 94–5
birth weight, low 66
blood
    clotting 10–11, 35, 36, 75, 76, 91,
        117, 118
    donors 107
    glucose levels 45–6, 49, 51, 54, 67,
        110, 113
    sugar levels 49, 50, 51, 110, 113
blood pressure 5, 7, 43, 77, 81, 85
    and alcohol 78
    checking 136
    effects of multinutrients *Fig 2*
    and exercise 74
    high (hypertension) 5, 10–12, 46, 49,
        66, 74–5, 83, 93, 101, 103–6, 122,
        131

ideal 11–12
    and magnesium 63
    and smoking 75, 135
blood vessels 8–11

caffeine 113
calcified valves 3
calcium 6, 63–4, 79, 100, 103–5, 133
cancer 95, 121
capillaries 8
carbohydrates 47, 51, 52–3, 76, 112
cardiovascular disease
    definition 14
    development 69–70
cardiovascular system 8–10, *Fig 1*
cells, rebuilding 138–9
cerebral haemorrhage 16
cerebrovascular disease 14
chest pain 16
cholesterol 5, 16, 18–26, 41, 49, 56, 85
    and garlic 117–18
    how body transports *Fig 4*
    ideal levels 22
    low level 24
    and magnesium 63
    and soya 109
    and vitamin C 39
chromium 53
claudication 16, 91
Co-Enzyme Q10 120–3, 137
coffee 47, 76–7, 83, 112–13, 127, 135
congenital defects 16
coronary artery disease 14, 42
coronary artery spasm 61, 62
coronary bypass operation 42, 61
cortisol 135
cystanthionine 56, 58

dairy products 29, 46, 51, 63, 70, 77,
    104, 109, 127
DHA (docosahexaenoic acid) 30, 32,
    79, 99, 100
diabetes 35, 41, 46, 48, 66, 67, 76, 83
diabetic angiopathy 41
diet 4, 6, 69–70, 72, 73, 76–80, 108–23
    and beta-carotene 95
    and calcium 105